WHAT YOUR
ACHES AND PAINS
ARE TELLING YOU

"A much-needed book for the 21st century; Odoul takes an energetic approach to holistic philosophy and goes to the root of energetic disturbances that lead to ailments or chronic conditions. Odoul connects us to the profound unconscious components of our minds and bodies to reconstruct physical ailments and thus develop transparency throughout our physical and our spiritual lives."

SEBHIA MARIE DIBRA, COAUTHOR OF *OVERCOMING ACUTE AND CHRONIC PAIN: KEYS TO TREATMENT BASED ON YOUR EMOTIONAL TYPE*

"In *What Your Aches and Pains Are Telling You,* Odoul demonstrates how pain tells your mind what is happening in your body, not only where, but why. He shows the reader how understanding your pain can provide pathways to healing."

MARC S. MICOZZI, M.D., PH.D., COAUTHOR OF *OVERCOMING ACUTE AND CHRONIC PAIN: KEYS TO TREATMENT BASED ON YOUR EMOTIONAL TYPE*

WHAT YOUR ACHES AND PAINS ARE TELLING YOU

Cries of the Body, Messages from the Soul

MICHEL ODOUL

Translated by Jack Cain

Healing Arts Press
Rochester, Vermont • Toronto, Canada

Healing Arts Press
One Park Street
Rochester, Vermont 05767
www.HealingArtsPress.com

Healing Arts Press is a division of Inner Traditions International

Originally published in French under the title *Dis-moi où tu as mal, je te dirai pourquoi: Les cris du corps sont des messages de l'âme*
First U.S. edition published in 2018 by Healing Arts Press

Note to the reader: This book is intended as an informational guide. The remedies, approaches, and techniques described herein are meant to supplement, and not to be a substitute for, professional medical care or treatment. They should not be used to treat a serious ailment without prior consultation with a qualified health care professional.

Library of Congress Cataloging-in-Publication Data

Names: Odoul, Michel, author.
Title: What your aches and pains are telling you : cries of the body,
    messages from the soul / Michel Odoul ; translated by Jack Cain.
Other titles: Dis-moi oáu tu as mal, je te dirai pourquoi. English
Description: First U.S. edition. | Rochester, Vermont : Healing Arts Press,
    2018. | Includes index.
Identifiers: LCCN 2017022512 (print) | LCCN 2017031360 (e-book) |
    ISBN 9781620556757 (paperback) | ISBN 9781620556764 (e-book)
Subjects: LCSH: Mind and body therapies. | Alternative medicine. | BISAC:
    HEALTH & FITNESS / Alternative Therapies. | BODY, MIND & SPIRIT / Healing
    / Energy (Chi Kung, Reiki, Polarity). | MEDICAL / Holistic Medicine.
Classification: LCC RC489.M53 O3413 2018 (print) | LCC RC489.M53 (e-book) |
    DDC 615.8/52—dc23
LC record available at https://lccn.loc.gov/2017022512

Printed and bound in the United States by P. A. Hutchison Company

10 9 8 7 6 5 4 3 2 1

Text design by Priscilla Baker and layout by Debbie Glogover
This book was typeset in Garamond Premier Pro with Arno Pro, Gill Sans MT Pro, and
Myriad Pro used for display fonts
Artwork by the author

To send correspondence to the author of this book, mail a first-class letter to the author c/o Inner Traditions • Bear & Company, One Park Street, Rochester, VT 05767, and we will forward the communication, or contact the author directly at his website, **www.shiatsu-institut.fr** (website in French but click on the British flag on the home page to find some English pages), or email him at **institutfrancaisdeshiatsu@wanadoo.fr**.

No man can reveal to you anything other than that which already lies half asleep in the dawning of your knowledge.

KAHLIL GIBRAN

◆ ◆ ◆

To the inner master who knows so well how to inspire us when we let life live and breathe within us

Contents

PART 1
A Philosophy of Human life
Energetic Connections Inside and Outside the Body

PART 2
A Symbolic Message System
How the Nonconscious Speaks through the Body

Foreword

The premise of Western medicine is that a given genetic foundation predisposes you to specific illnesses. The predisposition can be congenital* or it can be acquired.† In Eastern traditions, however, illness always indicates an obstacle in the accomplishment of one's Life Path. This is how the nonconscious, using energetic disturbances that can eventually lead to illness, speaks to us about what is hindering our full spiritual development and evolution. These two approaches are not necessarily incompatible (especially when we know, for example, that under stress mice can develop chromosome mutation). That's why, even when given exactly the same genetics, one person can develop an illness and the other remains in good health.

Instead of venturing into complex and hazardous genetic manipulation, it seems simpler—more reasonable and less costly—to restore health by understanding the psychoenergetic mechanisms that underlie illness. That is why Michel Odoul's book is a practical manual for anyone wanting to discover the keys to deciphering the body's language. In reading it, perhaps we may learn to no longer see illness as something caused by chance or fate or some external source outside of oneself, but instead to see it as a message from the nonconscious, from one's inner being, what

---

*Based on one's human leukocyte antigen, or HLA, a complex of genetically determined antigens occurring on the surface of almost every human cell by which one person's cells can be distinguished from another's
†Through chromosome mutation

Michel Odoul calls the "inner master." By taking this approach we will discover how behind our aches and pains lies a "creative illness" in the sense of pointing to a means of moving forward in one's spiritual evolution.

By simply and clearly revealing the psychoenergetic mechanisms that govern the organization of the macrocosm and the microcosm according to the Taoist approach, the author leads us toward discovering the deeper meaning of our aches, pains, and illnesses based on where the symptom is located in the body. For a long time this has been a vast area of inquiry for me, one that is rarely investigated or is muddied by contradictory conclusions. This book clarifies my own perceptions about the underlying causes of illness while providing an invaluable guide that can be used in any medical setting. These perceptions are given even more validation in that they are in harmony with Western psychological traditions, as has been shown by French psychotherapist Annick de Souzenelle, for example.

Odoul's approach, however, is based on two necessary and related conditions: that we take full responsibility for our own state of health and well-being, and that we give up the popular image of the all-powerful doctor as some sort of a savior. These conditions are the price for gaining a fully meaningful life.

This book can be quite useful to medical doctors and other practitioners who want to expand their awareness of illness beyond the simple mechanistic approach in order to assist each patient in understanding and realizing his or her own path. As the major objective of the twenty-first century resides in the reconciliation of opposites, perhaps we can envision a day when allopathic medicine, homeopathy, acupuncture, body-mind approaches, and the various forms of Eastern medicine (or at least the philosophical principles underpinning them) might coexist harmoniously.

THIERRY MÉDYNSKI, M.D.

Dr. Médynski, a medical doctor with specialties in homeopathy and psychology, is coauthor of the book *Psychanalyse et ordre mondial* (Psychoanalysis and World Order, published by Montorgueil). He currently works at an oncology facility in the south of France.

Note to the Reader

All the case studies in this book refer to real people; however, to maintain their privacy they are identified only by first names that are not their real names. Any resemblance to someone having that name and experiencing the same condition is a sign no doubt that what is written in this book is accurate, but in no case does it refer to that particular person.

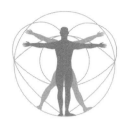

Introduction

We are living in times in which the tools of communication have never been as powerful, what with cell phones, laptops, and tablets that allow us to write, text, or speak to anyone in the world at any moment through the all-pervasive internet. However, this picture is not quite so rosy as it seems. Our communication is too often empty, vague, or misleading, only pretending to be real communication. All our gadgets are frequently only devices we use to compensate for our inability to have real, meaningful exchanges with others.

The way we conduct our lives, what with the pervasiveness and power of the media, the trap of materialism, and the accelerated pace of daily life, has gradually led us to believe that merely existing is living, that agitation and frenzy is energy. This has happened with our implicit consent. In fact, we even ask for it—always more, always faster; that's how we feel. But to what end? Is it to wake up one day at whatever age, sick and depressed, only to realize that we have missed out on life?

We have been conditioned by modern society to try to satisfy our desires through external means, so we have learned how to manage, master, control, and communicate with what is outside of us. Every day this rat race takes us further from our true, authentic self, eating away at our essence. It is only death or illness that seems to bring us back, forces us back, to face ourself. And when this happens, as it inevitably does, we feel helpless. Who is this unfamiliar person we sadly discover in the mirror? What does it mean that this body hurts? Who is this almost total stranger languishing in bed? And yet this stranger is our first and only true self, the one we've never *really* spoken to or taken the time to get to know. Discovering this unfamiliar self can be so disturbing that we'll ask the doctor to give us whatever it takes to silence the suffering that we reject. And yet, if we only knew! The issues that underlie pain and suffering are nothing more than desperate cries for recognition that our life and our body are sending us. They are warning signs, indications that we are out of balance with our true nature, but all too often we are unable to hear these warnings, much less understand them.

This book proposes to mitigate this deficiency by helping us open to the messages that our body is sending us when we are in pain. In this book we will position the human being in terms of the structures of life so we can understand how to embark on the path of wholeness. We will be studying the rules of functioning and the reasons behind this incredible game called life. We are going to learn to recognize and understand pain, tension, and suffering so that we can do what we need to do to bring ourself back into harmony and balance.

After many years of practicing energy techniques, specifically shiatsu, I have been able to realize to what extent, for each one of us, our body speaks to us (shouting even) about what we are really experiencing in the depths of ourself. Our deepest reality, our nonconscious, our mind, our soul—whatever your preferred term is—speaks to us constantly, telling us what isn't working. But we don't listen and we don't understand. Why? The reasons are twofold. First, we are not able or we don't want to listen to the messages sent to us through our dreams, intuitions, premonitions, physical sensations, and so forth. So these messages become stronger and stronger (in the form of illnesses, accidents, conflicts, etc.) so we can finally pay attention and stop doing what is causing us to be out of balance. The second reason why we don't pay attention to what our body is really saying is that even though we cannot, most of the time, avoid perceiving pain, we don't know how to decipher it or read it. So the pain may stop the maladjusted process for a while, but we don't radically change what has brought it about. No one has ever taught us how to make sense of pain. Our modern dualistic science separates the body from the mind and spirit. Science looks at the body, dissects it and studies as if it was a machine, while our doctors are, for the most part, good mechanics at best. We are like sailors receiving messages in Morse code yet we never learned the language of Morse code, so the incessant *beep-beep* of pain ends up being unpleasant. It bothers us, upsets us. So we call the mechanic onboard to block the system or, worse still, cut the wire to silence the noise, bringing us a kind of temporary relief. The thing is, that *beep-beep* is trying to warn us that there's a crack in the hull of the ship that's in need of caulking.

This is the coded language that we are going to learn to decipher in this book. And because it doesn't seem right to simply fire off indications that if it hurts in such and such a spot then it has such and such a meaning, I explain *why* it works that way. That is why this book is organized in two parts. In the first part I present the overarching, holistic philosophy that explains how everything is an interconnected whole. By knowing this we can better understand the reasons behind the "choice" of a certain pain or illness, because we will be connecting the mind, the soul, and the conscious and nonconscious with the physical body that experiences pain.

Here I draw on the Taoist codification of energies—specifically the concept of yin and yang and the energy meridians we know about from acupuncture—to show where a person fits within his or her energy environment.

In the second part of this book I conduct a "house inspection," providing a simple explanation of the role of each part and organ of the body. Finally, I show what effects are produced by what causes. In other words, I will provide you with a key to the symbolism of the body's messages.

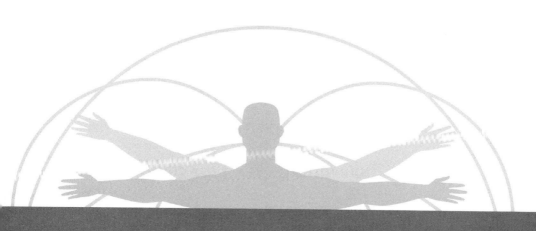

PART 1

A Philosophy of Human Life
Energetic Connections Inside and Outside the Body

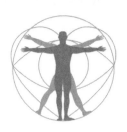

1

The Spiritual Dimensions of Human Life

Underpinnings of Our Being

> *He who has an appropriate concept of Providence doesn't stand beside a wall that is about to fall down.*
>
> MENCIUS

To understand the relationship between body and mind, and consequently the meaning of the body's ills in relation to the soul's bruises, we must enlarge the view we have of the human being and life itself. If we remain stuck in the materialist concept of man-as-machine, with its notion of the body as a series of independent, interchangeable parts, much like a car, then the subtle-energy connections that I am about to outline here are going to seem like magical thinking. Yet this is precisely the point—that the physical manifestations and symptoms of illness that we experience point to something deeper that lies within us.

Simple mechanical observation cannot reveal the true source of pain and illness because its view is too much glued to symptoms; the field of observation is limited in terms of both time and space. This prevents us from going to the real cause of our problems, which the mechanistic view explains in terms of fate (in the case of accidents) or interaction with external elements (in the form of viruses, microbes, food, or the environment). By expanding our view and observing the human being as a whole, both physically and temporally, we can begin to "connect the dots." This is what religion (from the Latin *religiare,* meaning "to connect" or "to link") was intended to do by assigning to humans a real dimension that is first and foremost spiritual. By taking this approach we can begin to understand humanity's mission and consequently the reasons for dis-ease.

The Process of Incarnation

According to Eastern tradition, life arises from chaos, as unformed magma, apparent disorder—facts that modern science and notably quantum physics are confirming today. Chaos is shaped through the action of a structuring force known as the Tao, which manifests as the two complementary forces of yin/Earth and yang/Heaven (see figure 1.1 on page 12). The human being is the meeting place of these two energetic expressions of the Tao. Initially coming out of chaotic magma, the human being is then no more than an energetic vibration without apparent form, which Taoists call the prenatal *Shen,* which corresponds to the terms *spirit* or *soul.* To exist, this Shen chooses to find support in the yin vibrations of a woman (the mother) and the yang vibrations of a man (the father). The subtle mixture of these three energies (Shen + energy of the mother + energy of the father) allows the human being to incarnate, that is, to exist in a physical body.

The process of incarnation is of course much more elaborate. I will explain more extensively how this takes place on an energetic level, but for the time being this simple explanation is enough for us to understand the following concepts.

The Life Path

The Life Path is a kind of connecting thread that each human being follows during the course of his or her life. Brazilian novelist and visionary Paulo Coelho uses the term *Personal Legend* in his beautiful book *The Alchemist* to describe the same thing. We can compare it to the script for a film or the "route map" for present-day rally enthusiasts. We move forward on this path by making use of the vehicle that is our physical body.

Here Eastern wisdom offers us a useful metaphor: the physical body is a carriage that travels down a path that symbolizes life—what I call the Life Path. The road on which the carriage travels is a dirt road. Like all unpaved roads it has potholes, bumps, stones, ruts, and ditches on both sides. The holes, bumps, and stones are the difficulties, the blows of life. The ruts are already existing patterns that we pick up from others and repeat in our own life. The ditches, some deep, some shallow, represent the rules, the boundaries that we have to stay within to avoid accidents. The road sometimes has low-visibility turns, and there can be areas of mist and storms that occlude the path. These are the times in life when we're "in the fog," where we have difficulty seeing or foreseeing clearly because we can't see what lies ahead. The carriage is pulled by two horses, one white (yang) on the left and one black (yin) on the right. The horses symbolize our emotions, which pull us around or even lead us through life. The carriage is driven by a coachman who represents our thinking mind, the conscious part of ourself. The carriage has four wheels. The front wheels correspond to our arms and maintain the direction, or rather convey the direction given by the coachman to the horses; the back wheels correspond to the legs, which carry and convey the load (and are therefore always bigger than the front wheels). Inside the carriage there is a passenger whom we don't see. This passenger is the inner master or guide, which each one of us has. This is the nonconscious or the holographic consciousness; Christians call it the guardian angel.*

---

*The nonconscious is a broader concept than the unconscious of Western psychology. It is the second part of human consciousness, which consists of two parts, one that is "conscious" and one that is not "conscious." The conscious part is the one we use for reflection, voluntary actions, work, and so on. The nonconscious part is the one that functions unconsciously, all the time. It is analogous to the prenatal Shen of Taoist

The carriage travels on life's road, apparently driven by the coachman. I say "apparently" because although he is certainly the driver, it is the passenger who has given the driver the destination. We will return to this explanation later in discussing the concept of the Earlier Heaven and the nonconscious as well as the choices made by the prenatal Shen and subsequently by the incarnated Shen. The coachman, which is our mind, our thinking process, drives the carriage. The quality and comfort of the trip (i.e., one's existence) depends on the quality of the coachman's attentiveness and how he drives (firmly but gently). If he mistreats the horses (the emotions) and bullies them, they will become agitated or bolt, possibly causing an accident, just as our emotions sometimes cause us to do unreasonable or even dangerous things. If the driver is too laid-back, if he lacks attentiveness, the team of horses will get into the ruts (in the form of replaying parental patterns, for example). Then we are following other people's footsteps and may end up in the ditch if that's what happened to them. In the same way, if he's not watchful the coachman is not going to be able to avoid dips, bumps, and potholes (blows, mistakes in life), so the trip will be very uncomfortable for the carriage, the coachman, and the inner master. If the coachman nods off or doesn't hold the reins, it will be the horses that end up driving the carriage. If the black horse is stronger (because we looked after him better), the carriage will veer to the right and be guided by maternal emotional representations. If the white horse is dominant because we have looked after him better, the carriage will veer to the left, toward paternal emotional representations. If the coachman drives too fast or pushes too hard, as we sometimes do, or if the horses bolt, it will be the ditch or an accident that will bring the conveyance to a stop more or less violently and with a certain amount of damage (accidents and trauma).

Sometimes a wheel or a part of the carriage gives way (sickness), either because it was weak or because the carriage hit too many bumps

---

(*cont.*) philosophy, which has chosen to incarnate in a particular human body because it is aware of what this particular soul needs to accomplish on Earth in this incarnation, that is, it knows the destination of the person's Life Path.

or too many potholes (behavioral overload, deficient attitudes). Then repairs will be needed, and depending on the seriousness of the breakdown we will either take care of it ourself (rest, regeneration), or we will call a handyman (alternative or natural medicine) or a mechanic (modern allopathic medicine). In any case, it will not be enough to just change the part. It's essential to think carefully about how the coachman drives and how we are going to change our behavior and the attitudes we have toward life if we don't want another breakdown.

Sometimes the carriage goes through zones where we can't see ahead clearly. There might be a turn in the road. We can see it coming so we have to slow down and check out the direction of the turn, following its curve, keeping the horses under control (mastering our emotions when we experience a time of deliberate or unexpected change). When there's fog or a storm it's harder to drive the carriage, so we must really slow down and pay attention to the sides of the road. At such times we need to have full or even blind confidence in the road ahead (the natural laws or the rules of the various traditions and religions); we must also have faith in the inner master (the nonconscious) that has chosen this road. These are the times in life when we are "lost in the fog," when we no longer know where we're going. At such times all we can do is let life show us the way.

Sometimes, as it happens, we come to a crossroads. If the road is not well marked we won't know what direction to take. The coachman (the thinking mind, the intellect) may pick a direction randomly. The more confident the coachman is, sure that he knows everything and has mastered everything, the more he will think he knows which direction to choose. In such cases the risks are proportionately greater. This is the realm of the "rational technocrat," where we believe that reason and the intellect alone can solve everything. On the other hand, if the coachman is humble and honest with himself he will ask the passenger, the inner master, which route to take. The passenger knows where he is going; he knows the final destination. He can then tell the coachman, who will take that direction on condition that the coachman is actually able to hear him. In fact, because the carriage sometimes makes a lot of noise as it rolls along, the coachman may need to stop the carriage to allow for an exchange with the master inside. These are the pauses, the time-outs that we sometimes take to reconnect with ourself, because it often happens that we lose contact with our own inner guidance, the inner knowledge of our own Life Path and destination.

So here we have a simple image that represents quite accurately what the Life Path is. This metaphor explains the way things happen in life and what can get us off track. Now I'm going to expand this discussion by looking at the concepts of the Earlier Heaven, the Later Heaven, and the conscious and nonconscious, as they also comprise the structure of the Life Path.

Earlier Heaven
and Later Heaven

Taoist philosophy says that there are two planes or dimensions to human life. The first is the one that precedes a person's birth, and the second is the one after his or her birth. In fact, birth marks the crossing of the threshold between these two "Heavens," as they are called in Taoism. Earlier Heaven represents everything that "is" or happens before birth—that is, before the moment when a human being appears in our world. Later Heaven refers to everything that "is" or happens afterward until death. Figure 1.1 on page 12 helps us visualize this better.

Earlier Heaven

What takes place at this level? What's in play at this stage? Earlier Heaven represents the phase of preexistence, where the prenatal Shen exists and is structured. Shen is equivalent to our Western concept of a soul. Earlier Heaven corresponds to the world of the infinite because

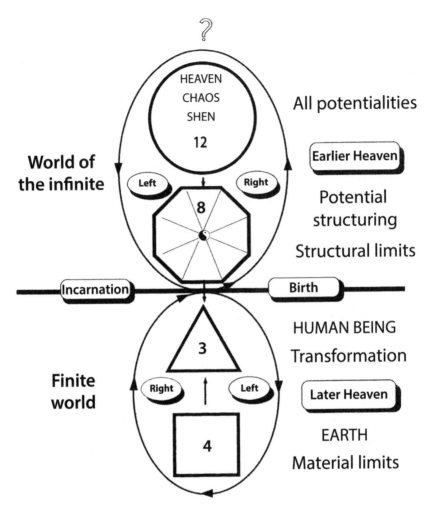

Fig. 1.1. Earlier Heaven and Later Heaven

there are no limits in either time or space. It carries within it all potentialities for life and is represented by a circle (any point on the circle is equally distant from the center). Here we find ourself at the level of chaos, the original magma. A person's prenatal Shen belongs to the Earlier Heaven as a drop of water belongs to the ocean; it keeps its individual consciousness the same way a drop of water always remembers that it belongs to the whole.

To illustrate this consciousness I like to use the concept of the hologram. In a hologram each point is positioned in a coherent way (as light) because it "knows" that it carries within itself all the information, the complete memory of all the other points. This is why I use the term *holographic consciousness* to describe Shen. We can find this holographic consciousness at the most subtle level of a human being. It helps us better understand how cellular growth can be managed from the egg to a full human (or animal), as well as the ongoing process of cellular renewal. It allows us to put forward an intriguing hypothesis regarding the extraordinary mysteries of self-healing available in the human body, as well as the possibility for illnesses such as cancer, autoimmune diseases, or AIDS.

The aim of each individual Shen is to realize its Life Path or Personal Legend, and for that it has to experience all existential polarities in order to transcend them and become a realized being. We all have our labors of Hercules. The limits of the manifest world (time, space, matter) do not allow for us to simultaneously live through all potentialities. They must be taken up through experience. The Shen must incarnate; that means it must learn in the school of life. And just as in school certain classes or lessons can sometimes be difficult to integrate, accept, or even understand, so the Shen has to try again and again. It does this by reincarnating, picking up the lesson at the point where it left off. This is the principle of reincarnation and the premise of karma. We will see later, by the way, that an equivalent principle called the repetition of patterns exists for the Later Heaven, in which a person who hasn't understood a previous mistake or false attitude will find himself behaving the same erroneous way again in exactly the same sort of situation until he can integrate the lessons that the situation has to offer.

Let's review the basic concept of karma because I believe it is sometimes explained in a very misleading way. Karma involves an evolutionary concept of life and is decidedly not a punitive philosophy as certain people would have us believe. These folks have been programmed by their Judeo-Christian cultural conditioning. We do not come back to expiate, pay off, or submit to the punishment of past bad behavior. All that is Manichean and in no way corresponds to the energetic paradigm that we are referring to, in which concepts of good and evil do not exist. This erroneous way of thinking about karma has no historical meaning anyway since concepts about values and what constitutes good and bad change according to the prevailing era, traditions, and culture. The principle of karma is much simpler and is based on the necessity for experimentation and integration of all of life's potentials. The school of life proceeds in the same way as all schools do, which is to say with classes, recreation periods, and lessons to learn and understand until they have been fully integrated.

As well there are also consequences for inappropriate behavior (that is, if we don't respect the rules of the game, if we conduct ourselves badly). Bills must be paid, so to speak. This is where the confusion around karma and its conflation with punishment comes up. Paying a bill doesn't mean punishment. A bill means that for every cause there is an effect, for every behavior there is a result, and if the behavior is not in harmony with the rules of how things work it will produce a result that is not satisfactory or pleasant. Let's take some simple examples: If we want something sweet, we know that a pastry will give us that sweetness. We eat it and indeed our craving for sugar is satisfied. Similarly, if we are near a hotplate and our hands are cold, we can warm them with the hotplate. But we also know that a hotplate can burn us and that we need to keep our distance from it. If we're in a hurry and want our hands to warm up faster and we get too close to the hotplate, the bill for this decision will be a burn. The burn is then in no way a punishment, but simply the result of inappropriate behavior in not respecting one of the criteria of the situation. The process with karma is exactly the same on a psychological level. There is no punishment in it—no sanction is set up, decided, and applied by someone or something that is external or transcendent. It is simply the effect, the logical result of a given behavior. In this case, the behavior was not in harmony with the laws of the context, and as a result there is a negative bill to pay—a burn and associated suffering. In the case of the pastry, the behavior of buying it is in harmony and produces a positive consequence, which is the satisfying of the desire for something sweet. However, if the behavior of eating sweets becomes excessive (compulsive), harmony with natural laws is lost and the behavior produces a negative bill, which would be weight gain and perhaps tooth decay.

Let's now return to the discussion of the Earlier Heaven. How do things take place? The Shen decides to incarnate to realize its Life Path, and in that way to learn a lesson from the life chosen. For this lesson to be learned there must be the means to make it happen. The Shen's choice will be made in relation to the given aim, the work that needs to be done, and also in relation to what has already been experienced and integrated and doesn't need to be repeated. All of this earlier (as in previous lifetimes) data is recorded in the Akashic Records, a sort of inner mythology consisting of holographic memories that each one of us has. The Taoists call them "old memories" or "early memories." To have a way of experiencing new potentialities, the Shen will choose structures and limits that will allow it to experience its choices under the best conditions, that is, the most favorable and also the most effective.

The concept of what constitutes effectiveness is formidable since it is far from meaning comfortable or pleasant. Here we touch on a crucial point in describing the Life Path. In fact, as we have seen earlier, all roads can have ditches or turns in which the vehicle of our existence experiences jolts or moments where there is a lack of visibility, in the same way that all Life Paths unfold through tests and ordeals. These are factors that astrology, and in particular karmic astrology, can help us grasp. The selection of conditions for achieving something allows us to bring together all the physical and environmental factors needed in an incarnation. Era, family, country, region, sex, race, and so forth then become the structural framework of the incarnation, and this provides us with the material limits we need for the Shen to incarnate.

Later Heaven

With incarnation we leave the plane of Earlier Heaven and move on to the Later Heaven. The prenatal Shen is attracted to a support medium (the fertilized egg) that corresponds to its vibratory frequency, to the conditions it needs in order to realize its Life Path. It is then added to the energies of the parents who have just fertilized this magical egg that will become a human being. These energies are in turn added to the environmental energies (planets, place, era, etc.) to form the individual Shen. The Shen, still inactive in the embryonic state, will continue to enrich itself by harvesting information right up to the moment of birth, to the cutting of the cord, when it actually becomes active. This is why astrological charts are calculated from the moment of birth and not from the date of conception.

How do things happen at the level of the Later Heaven? Here we are at the level of the finite world. Limits are imposed by the material, tangible world. The incarnated being experiences existence through a physical body and certain material constraints. The survival of this body implies a certain number of rules and obligations that are both universal (eating, drinking, sleeping) and local (culture, place, climate). These limits impose a very precise functioning on the person and correspond to the fulfillment of this particular choice of incarnation. The newly arrived human being's physical reality, the body, is completely subject to the constraints of this framework, whereas his or her psychological and emotional realities are a little less constrained by it.

These material limits are support points on which our realization rests and are that through which the realization is carried out and manifests itself. Because of this, these limits can, conversely, be a remarkable means for deciphering and understanding the part that we play in the things that manifest within us. This is true for our body, for our emotions, for our psychology, for our environment, and for everything that "happens to us." What we have in our material limits is an extraordinary tool for knowledge—all the more reason to try to decipher them.

The Concept of Laterality

As we can see from figure 1.1, we have in the Earlier Heaven and the Later Heaven a right and a left. However, we can see that they are reversed. This touches on an important decoding element in our study: laterality. This reversal allows us to understand why psychomorphology* and modern psychology position within the human body the connection to the mother on the left side of the body and the connection to the father on the right side of the body, whereas traditional Chinese medicine and Taoist philosophy do the reverse. This can be explained by the fact that the West has always been much more preoccupied with the unmanifest aspects of a being—the spirit and the soul, those elements that come from the Earlier Heaven— rather than with the body and physical, material reality, which are considered "lower" and belong to the Later Heaven. The East, on the other hand, has always been preoccupied with the here and now, with real experience in the present moment, with the manifest aspects, the elements that come from the Later Heaven. So the physical body and material reality are very important to the East since it is through them that the Shen expresses itself.

The West bases its approach then on elements that belong mainly to the Earlier Heaven, whereas the East bases its approach mainly on the Later Heaven, at least for physical laterality. This is why they are reversed in the Later Heaven. It is similar to what takes place with the image of reality that the eye perceives that in turn is transmitted to and interpreted by the brain. For the East, the right side of the body is related to yin and consequently to maternal symbolism, while the left side is related to yang and to paternal symbolism. This specificity is extremely important to our discussion because the physical laterality of

---

*The word *psychomorphology* is derived from two Greek words, *psyche,* meaning "soul," and *morphos,* meaning "shape, shade, size." Psychomorphology argues that behavior to a large extent is a product of inbred, congenital, inherited, ingrained, inborn nature, structure, and formation, and this in turn is responsible for a person's personality.

symptoms and traumas are elegant and revealing descriptions of what takes place in our depths. Given that these manifestations belong to what is manifest and therefore to the Later Heaven, they are codified by the lateralization proposed by the East (right = maternal symbolism). Conversely, everything that takes place in a person's psychology, in what is imagined, in dreams, or which took on a form before birth (psycho-morphology), belongs to the Earlier Heaven and corresponds therefore to the lateralization mainly used by the West.

Let's consider an example. A child who is born with a right ear slightly larger than the left ear is going to have a stronger relationship and a dependency on or favor listening to his father. Why? If the child is born with a larger ear it is because it was formed in this way *before* birth. It was structured in this form in the Earlier Heaven, in the unmanifest. At this level, the right is in relationship with the paternal symbolism and left with the maternal symbolism. Everything that comes from the father both educationally and culturally will be received and perceived with a greater sensitivity, a greater attention to listening, but doubtless also with a greater dependency.

If on the other hand, the child shows otitis (an ear infection) in this same right ear, we are in the manifest world, in the experience of the child after his birth. The right ear is then in relation to the maternal symbolism, for we are in the Later Heaven, in what is manifest. It is the child who has set in motion a symptomatic manifestation in his present-day physical body after his birth. Here, laterality reverses and the right enters into relationship with the maternal symbolism. The otitis means that he doesn't want to hear what comes from his mother, that his listening to what comes from her does not satisfy him. Perhaps she shouts too much or she constantly tells him things like "Be careful, don't do that, you're going to fall, you'll hurt yourself," or "Don't catch cold," and so forth.

Here's another example: the case of a person who *dreams* she sprains her left ankle. Although this incident took place after birth, we are nevertheless in this case in the unmanifest, the virtual, since it took place in the oneiric world, the world of dreams. This particular sprain then needs to be considered in relation to its maternal symbolism. In contrast, if this person really does sprain her left ankle, we are in the manifest. Then the sprain has a symbolically paternal meaning and could express, for example, a problem of status or an attitudinal issue with a man.

Given the importance of this concept of laterality, we can synthesize what we've just covered in the following table:

	Before birth	After birth	
	Formation of the body	Trauma, illness, symptoms	Alpha states, premonitions, dreams
Right side of the body	Paternal symbolism	Maternal symbolism	Paternal symbolism
Left side of the body	Maternal symbolism	Paternal symbolism	Maternal symbolism

The Conscious and the Nonconscious

What can we be aware of? Going back to figure 1.1 and comparing to figure 1.2 on page 20, we can see that the Earlier Heaven becomes the nonconscious, the nighttime consciousness and inner silence, while the Later Heaven becomes the conscious, the daytime consciousness and the phenomenal and external.

The Nonconscious

We know that the Earlier Heaven represents the level of preexistence, the stage where existence is prepared on all planes (rules, structures, choices, etc.). When we switch at the time of incarnating, the Earlier Heaven becomes the nonconscious. This nonconscious then represents the premanifest, or the level at which the manifest is prepared (the manifest being what happens in the tangible, conscious world). Acts, actions, accomplishments, and so forth are the domain of the manifest. They are what we can perceive, and they may be directly associated with

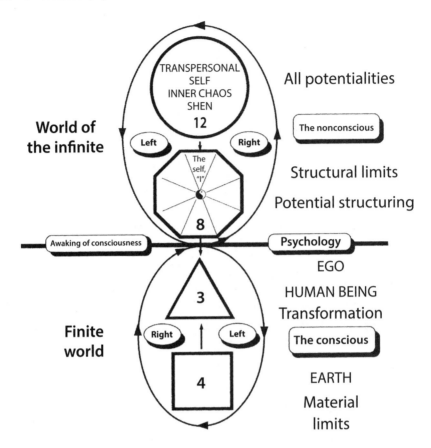

Fig. I.2. The conscious and the nonconscious

horizontality, that is, with all things concerning the material dimension of life. However, they are first "prepared" in the nonconscious.

The holographic consciousness that I spoke of earlier is located in the nonconscious. It is what deploys the actions that allow us to materialize our choices in carrying out our Life Path. This holographic consciousness carries within it the memory and knowledge of the inner choices that we have made in the Earlier Heaven; it knows the totality of our Akashic Record, our personal mythology. The nonconscious has at its disposal all of this information; consequently it knows the ramifications of our choices; it knows our need to experiment in order to learn our life lessons, and it also can determine the best choices, those that will allow us to succeed in life. It is here that confusion can arise around the concepts of freedom, determinism, destiny, fate, and inevitability. If the processes are observed after the fact and without stepping back, it could be said, "It is written" (i.e., fated). It was indeed written, but not in the sense in which we follow a script established by something or someone outside ourself, where we are mere puppets animated or directed by some external force. Indeed, it *is* written, but only in the sense that *we* write it. In other words, we write within ourself, within our nonconscious, the best possible script for achieving the chosen aim.

We can perhaps understand this more easily with an image. If, for example, I want to go to a fair in Chicago, this will lead me to make logistical choices that fulfill my aim. First of all I have to set aside some vacation time and reserve a hotel room in Chicago for that period of time. My preferences will of course influence my choice of hotel. If, on the other hand, I don't have much experience in this kind of thing I might not know that I have to make my hotel reservations well in advance; otherwise I risk not finding a hotel room. Then I have to decide how to get there. If I like driving and I'm not in a hurry I might decide to drive. If beautiful countryside is something that interests me, I might choose the backroads instead of the highways. In that case I should definitely leave a day earlier. If I dread driving I might take a train, and if I'm in a hurry I might fly. This example shows how what is already within us conditions our choices. To attain a given aim, each person proceeds according to his or her own choices, in a manner conditioned by the nonconscious.

That said, once the decision has been made I'm free at any time to change my mind and not go to Chicago. Or if I do there's nothing to stop me from getting off the train in Cleveland or Pittsburgh if I want to stop and see my relatives there if I'm going by car. On the other hand, if I fly, it's going to be harder to do that if it's a nonstop flight from New York to Chicago. The more last-minute my decision to change my plans is, the more that decision will cost me, but change is still possible.

However, if the aim of the side trips to Pittsburgh and Cleveland is to settle some difficult and unpleasant business with my relatives, my choice to go straight to the fair and avoid the difficult situation would mean that sooner or later—in this case later—I will have to face this situation. The more I put it off, the more difficult and costly—in terms of the unpleasantness that could arise from avoiding the situation—it will be for me.

However, if I've done everything appropriately and for the greater good, I will be in Chicago for the fair under the conditions that suit me. This might mean that despite my overriding desire to attend the fair, I feel guided to make those side trips because I know that resolving difficulties with my relatives will be good for all of us. This shows how our choices are conditioned by preexisting "memories"—in this case, I feel compelled by some inner urge to resolve old karmic ties with my relatives. This inner urgency is coming from my nonconscious need to resolve these difficulties, which may even go back to past lifetimes.

But let's suppose that someone from the outside—say, an extra-terrestrial who is not familiar with the customs and habits of Earthlings—is observing my choices. What does he see? He sees a person at the fair in Chicago. If he studies what took place before my arrival in Chicago, what does he notice? All my actions preceding my arrival (taking vacation time, making hotel and plane reservations, etc.) lead him to only one conclusion: everything got put together and unfolded so that I got to Chicago that day. He might then conclude that it was "written" that I should go to Chicago because all my actions have unfolded in such a way that it appears as if they had been predetermined, as if I am a puppet controlled by a puppeteer. This would be missing the point: that it is *I* who chose to go to Chicago, and no one else.

The whole fabric of our history is written in our prenatal Shen, in our holographic consciousness; its staging is conducted by our nonconscious, which is our inner master. To use our earlier metaphor, our conscious (the coachman) and our physical body (the carriage) are its visible and favored actors. They must respect the staging and their role, but they do have a certain freedom, the possibility of improvisation, which is conditioned by the basic path they are traveling. When everything unfolds according to the greater good, at the end of day—upon our death—we will have the satisfaction of knowing that we respected the path and successfully met life's challenges. Conversely, if we do not respect the path, then there is dissonance between the conscious and the nonconscious, a dissonance between the inner master, the coachman, and the carriage. This is when tension in the form of suffering, illness, accidents, and other slipups appear. In fact, it seems that the grand purpose of existence is for the conscious and the nonconscious—for the master, the coachman, and the carriage—to come into alignment. Here we find, I believe, the secret of profound harmony and true serenity that shows us to what an extent a congruent life is not the prerogative of a culture or an education but quite simply the result of individual work that is clear and uncompromising. It is why this concept of harmony is very distinct from the concepts of intellect or culture. It depends solely on the individual's level of cohesion among these elements: what he is, what he does, and his Life Path. It follows then that we can encounter and feel this profound strength in, for example, a Tibetan lama, a shepherd from Larzac, a schoolmarm in the far reaches of Cantal (I was born there), a Brittany fisherman, a modern philosopher, a biologist, or an old English gardener.

The Conscious

In the realm of the conscious, things appear little by little as they manifest gradually in a tangible way. This takes place in the person first at the level of the energies of the body, then at the level of the emotions (conscious emotions), and finally in the psychology (the conscious psychology). The process continues next to the physical level and manifests in the meridians, then in the organs, and finally in the limbs. At this point we come to the densest level of energy, at the level of Earth, the place where the material limits on us are the heaviest and the most constraining.

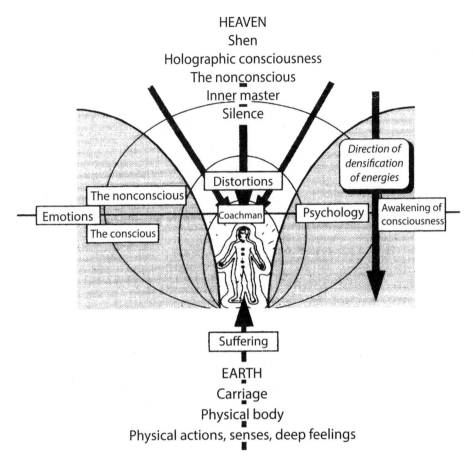

Fig. 1.3. The densification of energies

The process of densification operates exactly the same way as the natural phenomenon of rainfall. First, there is humidity in the air. This is usually not perceptible (nonconscious) except by very sophisticated equipment. After a certain amount of time and under certain conditions the humidity begins to densify, condensing into water vapor. It then forms clouds (ideas, thoughts, emotions, desires, intentions, etc.), which are perceptible although still without much consistency. Certain of these clouds are light and present no risk of a storm (emotions, thoughts, negative intentions). The water vapor continues to densify in

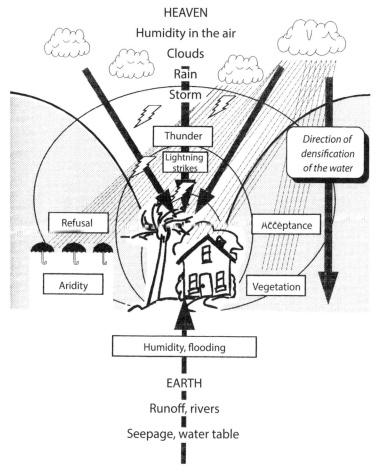

HEAVEN
Humidity in the air
Clouds
Rain
Storm

Thunder

Lightning strikes

Direction of densification of the water

Refusal

Acceptance

Aridity

Vegetation

Humidity, flooding

EARTH

Runoff, rivers

Seepage, water table

Fig. 1.4. The phenomenon of rainfall as a metaphor for awakening

clouds, finally producing drops of rainwater or even a storm. At this point rain then falls to the ground, the earth (our body), which gets wet from the water (deep feelings, tension, suffering). When the storm (tension) is strong, thunder rumbles and lightning sometimes may strike (heart attack, epileptic seizure, fainting, madness, etc.). This process is illustrated by figure 1.4 above, which should be compared to the previous figure, figure 1.3.

The shift between the nonconscious and the conscious takes place by awakening the consciousness. This awakening happens by moving into action, by doing, and it represents the last stage in the densification of energies. Through the results produced by doing we can realize where we stand and will have a "moment of awakening." If the result obtained is "good"—that is, if it fits with our higher purpose—it means that the process was coherent overall and that we have respected all the intermediate phases of the execution, whatever they may be. This process isn't, of course, completely conscious, and for that reason we sometimes have to make mistakes or suffer in order to understand just where things are not going our way. That is why I put the word *good* in quotation marks, because certain disagreeable experiences are in fact good for our spiritual evolution, like a violent thunderstorm that may be unpleasant but brings ample rain to moisten the earth, nourish plants, and make all of nature rejoice. Rejecting life's challenges, trying to insulate oneself from them, deprives a person of necessary experiences, just as a rain shield leads to aridity. Difficult experiences cause us to reflect about what is happening and no doubt lead to us making the changes necessary to help us grow—provided we are ready to listen to the underlying message. Otherwise we keep repeating the same old patterns until we finally understand what our experiences are trying to tell us and change our behavior.

The Process of Awakening

The nonconscious tries to speak to us about actions and behavior that are not in accord with our spiritual evolution. It tries to get our attention through physical, psychological, or emotional suffering. At first it sends preliminary messages; then it shouts and screams at us if we don't listen and are unable to figure out what in our behavior or thinking is discordant with our growth. It is therefore very important to understand the true meaning behind any pain, illness, and suffering if we really want true and deep healing. That's why the modern scientific/medical approach of fighting against these deep-seated expressions of our relationship to life in general and to our own life in particular will always be a losing battle. Life will always be one step ahead of us, and we will never manage (thank goodness!) to silence her, to muzzle her. The more medical science tries to treat an illness through a mechanistic model, the more such an illness becomes even more deep-seated, more difficult to handle, and more capable of mutating—because we are ignoring the deeper message behind the illness. It is so much better to try to understand what our pain and illness is trying to tell us instead of trying to silence it through pharmaceutical drugs or by enduring it, believing the religious dogma that teaches that suffering is obligatory, inevitable, and deserved because we are "sinners."

Can we can avoid suffering and illness? Yes, when we really search for new understanding. Even when facing death we can put our pain and suffering into a feedback process in which we look at what the pain is trying to tell us. Once the underlying causes of pain reach the dense physical level of expression, it is possible for pain to turn around and go in the opposite direction through a process of release and freedom. But this transformation can only take place if we don't block the densi-fied energies. By "killing" their expression by medicating ourself or by believing that we somehow deserve to suffer, as religious dogma tells us, we interrupt the all-important feedback loop. We prevent the underly-ing message of pain from moving back up, returning to its source on a more subtle level of the nonconscious, such that at the first opportunity the pain is going to manifest again, releasing not only the energy of ten-sion in that moment, in that context, but also the energy of all the pre-ceding situations that have not been freed up or that we have silenced.

We can return to the metaphor of rain, as shown in figure 1.5 on page 28, to more easily understand this process of liberation. The rain moistens the earth, and the earth gives the water back to the heavens by letting it flow naturally in rivers and streams into the sea. The water evaporates and transforms into water vapor and humidity, which pro-duces rainfall. This is the healthy cycle. If, on the other hand, the earth retains the water somehow (trapped underground, bottled up by a dam or reservoir), the places where it is imprisoned will fill up with each rain

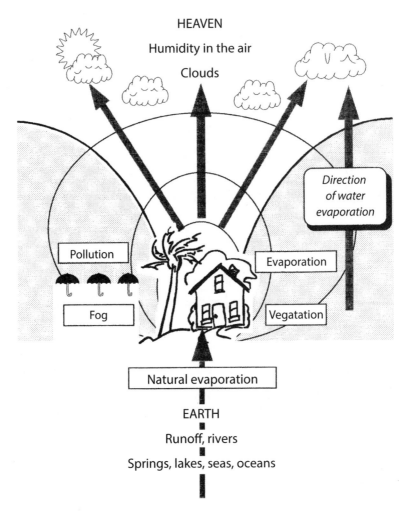

Fig. 1.5. The phenomenon of evaporation

shower to the point where if there is a strong storm in which the earth cannot absorb any more water, everything breaks: the dam gives way with devastating results, including landslides and flooding.

It's exactly the same for us. If we block the natural flow of our energy with our inner obstacles—the negative emotions of anger, bitterness, resentment, etc.—the tensions and the suffering remain within us and produce a boomerang effect that feeds on itself and darkens our daily life, just as air pollution creates a more and more opaque dome above

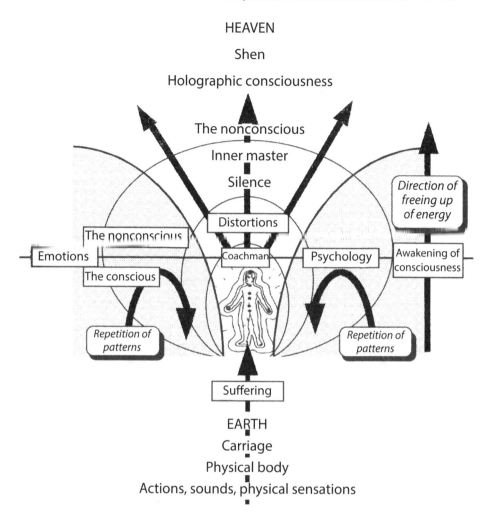

Fig. 1.6. Liberation, the freeing up of blocked energy

our cities. However, if we don't block these energies—notably, if we accept pain for what it means on a deeper level, if we even anticipate it in the form of recognizing our own obstacles within and in doing so avoid the need for it to appear outwardly as illness, the process of liberation, as seen in figure 1.6, is set in motion. This manifests on the physical level as relief from suffering and pain, an experience that truly feels like liberation or even a miracle. I do not believe there is anything other than this behind what are described as "miraculous" healings such as spontaneous remissions of cancer that seem so inexplicable by science.

Here I can't help but think about a spectacular example of this process of liberation that I once encountered. A young woman came to see me for relaxation work and harmonization of her energies. She was very tense and in pain as a result of a seriously herniated disc in the cervical vertebrae and was scheduled to undergo surgery. Locked in a neck brace with her face showing the effects of numerous sleepless nights, she was obviously going through a really hard time. After doing the initial work of harmonization we were able to get to the heart of her problem, what was really behind her physical suffering. First, I guided her in identifying what emotional trauma could be hidden behind the physical problem. Then we worked on trying to understand what that trauma could mean, how it got etched into her life, and what the real meaning of it was. What happened was astonishing. As we worked together, without this young woman realizing it, her neck gradually started to visibly let go as she spoke and allowed her tears to flow. More and more she began to move her head, turning it to such an extent that after a while I interrupted her to say, "Do you realize that you are moving your head perfectly normally, without any obvious impediment?" She stopped speaking for a few seconds then burst out laughing with tears still in her eyes. Her neck brace now served no purpose and neither did her pain. She understood and accepted the sense of the heavy ordeal that had struck her so long ago and she was able to erase the emotional memory that had remained stuck in her neck as severe pain.

Here is what's important: If she had gone ahead and gotten the surgery, which is what she had done to resolve a herniated disc at an earlier time, she would not have come to the deeper understanding of what had caused so much pain in her life. She would have gone through the pain of surgery without the deeper understanding behind it all, an understanding that resulted in her healing on the physical level.

This example shows how it is very important for us to accept pain as part of a process of discovery. If we can, to whatever extent possible, allow this process to unfold, it will reach a crisis point. Then with realization and understanding the process will shift, and the physical effects of the deeper issue will diminish and eventually completely disappear. This point of crisis cannot always be reached by everyone suffering from pain, but that's not what's most important. What's important is to go as far as we can in the process, each time making a little more headway. It's like training in sports—daily stretching opens up the muscles and joints and gradually makes the body more flexible. Daily work on pain as a process of discovery allows you to gradually open the body. But take care, all of this works in a healthy way only on condition that we act intelligently and not go too far, changing a developmental process into a new form of dysfunctional behavior.

The awakening of consciousness will help us in this by playing the role of "door-keeper." By working on the emotions, which exist on both the conscious and the nonconscious levels, we facilitate our own awakening. This awakening makes its way up to the level of the holographic consciousness, and once there it can choose new experiential modes. It is at this level that the person comes to the phase of acceptance, to the integration of the experience of those deeply felt emotions. This phase is difficult because it belongs to the conscious and present level in which the person continually reencounters existing feelings. Accepting these difficult emotions instead of pushing them away allows us to look at them in a new way as we integrate the deeper meaning of the experience. This in turn allows for forgiveness, which is fundamental and necessary to the process, as it conditions the shift toward the nonconscious. If this shift doesn't take place, the person falls back into the same old pattern, causing him or her to undergo the same physical experiences, often more strongly with each repetition, because the underlying message of the illness has not been accepted and understood. If this is the case, then the person is merely "keeping score" (with life, with others, with himself) instead of "closing the accounts." He is simply perpetuating the same old pattern. Such a person exists in a state of conflict, at war with his inner master, which takes him further and further away from balance, inner peace, and being at peace with life. On the other hand, if the shift is done correctly, the freeing process then moves into the plane of the nonconscious, where the work shifts to a deeper psychological level following the same logic as on the conscious plane, in dreams, for example. In this phase the person must go back to those old, deep inner wounds linked for instance to childhood in order to understand the memories of those hurts and try to sympathize with the emotions they bring up—that is, to accept them and recognize them for what they are, without judging them or struggling against them. It's at this level that the real letting go happens, the kind of letting go that occurs when life pushes us to the max. Here we are obliged to let go because to continue fighting against the momentum of the process is useless. There is nothing left to do but to accept what is taking place and forgive if necessary. This is the letting-go phase, the Christian "Thy will be done" and the Islamic "Inshallah." At no time is this an abandonment, an abdication; instead it represents an acceptance, an inner welcoming of the way things are that goes beyond our personal ego self. It is at this point that things change in astonishing ways, such that once-inextricable situations seem to turn around completely.

To pick up again the example of so-called spontaneous remission: These always occur in people who are in the final stages of cancer and have been diagnosed as terminal. Supposedly nothing more can save them. They have been told that they have very little time left and to get their affairs in order. It is at this moment that certain people shift into this last level, the stage of acceptance, of integration. In an astonishingly small amount of time (a few days in many cases), their bodies become completely healthy. With acceptance and integration of the deeper meaning of the illness, stagnant energy is freed up and memories of the past are rewritten, leaving room for new interpretations of old memories and choices. It is this final acceptance that facilitates the "miraculous" remission.

If we don't go through one of these letting-go stages when faced with difficulties, we must inevitably begin the process again until we do accept the reality of the situation. Of course it is clear that all these processes of discovery function continually, at all levels and with varying degrees of intensity, and not solely by causing serious illnesses or intense suffering. Most of the time they are nonconscious and it is only in difficult cases that they manifest with so much force. However, these processes will continually appear at our densest energetic level, that is, in our physical body. How does that take place and what are the favored means for these manifestations?

Physiological Expressions of Disharmony

Like all energetic realities in our world, human reality needs its medium of expression, the physical body, in order to be able to express what is taking place in the innermost reaches. It is clear that we all need gestures, words, or images to be able to express our ideas, thoughts, and feelings. All of these intangible phenomena would not exist, in the sense that they would not be perceived, if there were not this possibility of manifestation. It's much like the most advanced computer in the world, which would be useless without its peripheral components (monitor, keyboard, printer, scanner, and so forth). It seems then that the human mind would have little reason to exist without its materialized projection: the physical body.

Continuing with the example of the computer, there would be no point in it being powerful if its peripheral components couldn't express its power. It would not be useful either to have extraordinary peripherals if the memory and processing capacity were not up to speed, such as, for example, having a color printer if the display is only black and white. It is the same for the person who has to seek balance between body and mind. By looking at what the body expresses it is possible to decipher what is going on in the mind and spirit of the person. When the whole body-mind-spirit functions in a coherent way, physical reality is in harmony with the spiritual reality of the person, and there is health as a result. When there is an imbalance between these aspects, between the conscious and the nonconscious, between the actor and the script, danger signals are going to appear. There are three main types of signals, three ways of experiencing these inner messages of distortion in the body: as nervous tension; as physical or psychological trauma; and as physical or psychological illness.

Tension

The first type of signal comes in the form of tension and discomfort, for example, tension in the back, digestive problems, nightmares, and psychological malaise or depression. This is a fairly common way inner tension expresses itself. Here the nonconscious expresses imbalance or inner conflict in physiological or psychological terms, producing a feeling to express what is happening. This is the inner master who is knocking on the window of the carriage to alert the coachman and let him know something isn't right (wrong direction, uncomfortable or dangerous driving, fatigue, need to take stock). If the person is open and ready to hear and accept the message at the conscious level, she will make the necessary behavioral changes and the tension will disappear. The more she has worked on herself and is in harmony with herself and with the finer and more powerful aspects of herself (the nonconscious), the more sensitive and capable she will be in perceiving and receiving this first type of message and the more capable of understanding it. If she has arrived at a certain level of self-awareness she will even be able to anticipate these messages and avoid the possibility of tension even arising.

Unfortunately, most of us have a hard time being receptive to even this early stage of messages. There are numerous reasons for this, in particular our natural tendency to want to take the easy way out and our culture's dualistic approach that says that things just happen to us as a result of some external agent. This is how we develop deafness to what the nonconscious is trying to tell us. This first level of messages is nevertheless extraordinarily rich. Numerous signs come to us from our environment, notably from what we might call the "mirror effect," a subject I will come back to later.

Trauma

To make itself heard the nonconscious must sometimes resort to stronger signals, including trauma and illness. In terms of effectiveness, these are clearly more hard-hitting messages than mere tension and discomfort. Trauma and illness are always offset in time in relation to their source. The gap is proportional to the person's deafness, to his or her inability to hear the underlying message. This offset is greater for illness than it is for trauma and both are proportionately greater than mental and psychological tension. That is, the offset in time is greater in relation to the meaning being "refused," notably because it touches areas of strong sensitivity in the individual. When the difficult information touches on key, fundamental aspects of the person, its effects can even take place on different planes of consciousness and in different incarnations on Earth. That is, an unresolved situation from a past life can generate physical symptoms in a person's current life.

Trauma in the body and limbs, usually in the form of some sort of accident, is a second stage in the gradation of messages. Here the person, through her nonconscious, seeks a solution. The accident is therefore an active expression in the sense that it represents a double initiative on the part of the person experiencing it. First, it is a new message, more blatant than the previous type, but despite everything is still a mode of open communication. The inner master is knocking much harder on the carriage window and might even break it to make enough noise to force the coachman to listen. This stage can still allow for a change in the situation concerned because it appears during a process of densification or freeing up of energies. It indicates that the person must stop and obliges her to take stock and halt the dysfunctional dynamic in order to understand what's really going on, and then make changes.

However, trauma can also be an active attempt to stimulate and free up tension that has accumulated due to some inner distortion or imbalance in the person. This is why it never appears randomly. The shock, break, sprain, fracture, etc., is going to happen at a very precise place in the body in order to stimulate the energies that circulate at that point or to release energy blockages at that point, sometimes both at the same time. Thus trauma can provide us with information of great precision as to what is really happening. Spraining the right ankle, cutting the left thumb, displacing the third cervical vertebra, bumping the head—in each case there is a specific message as to what is wrong.

For example, in one of my seminars I was outlining this very idea and providing examples. I was talking about knee problems and explained that these problems indicate tension in relationship with others, and in particular difficulties in letting go of, bending to, or accepting something connected to a relationship with another person. I received a gigantic burst of laughter from someone in response. I addressed the person who had just expressed his disagreement to me in this way and asked him what was so funny in what I had just said. The man replied that he had sprained his knee two years earlier simply because he was competing in an intense soccer match and had kicked the ball while turning around. He asserted that there was nothing in that to understand except that in team sports you can get hurt. I asked him which knee he had injured. The right, he replied. I then suggested that he consider if at that point in time he was experiencing any tension in a relationship with a woman where he was refusing to let go of something. Not wanting to get sidetracked into a discussion at this point I went on to something else without asking him to reply. During the next half hour I observed him thoughtfully pondering my question. Suddenly his face began to turn shockingly white. I stopped to ask him what was going on. He then shared with the group what he had just remembered: The day before the match his wife had served him with a divorce proceeding. He had been in conflict with her for several months because he had refused to give her the divorce.

Trauma is active because it manifests in the yang element. It generally involves external parts of the body such as the limbs, the head, or the upper body. It acts at the level of defensive energies that circulate mainly on the surface of the body. The wounded part becomes an essential piece of information for understanding, but laterality provides even more precision as to the deeper meaning. A sprain of the wrist means something in general, but whether it's the right or the left will pinpoint the meaning even more accurately. You need to know that the stronger the tension is or the longer it lasts without being perceived, the more likely it is that the resulting trauma is great or even violent. Trauma is a positive signal in the sense that it represents an unconscious attempt, albeit extreme, to release, to change things. It is clear that the deeper message of trauma must be acknowledged and understood, otherwise we will fail to gain any insight.

Illness

The third type of message comes from illness, either physical or psychological. This involves the yin element in the sense of representing what is occurring in the depths of the body or the mind. The person is eliminating tension, but in this case in a "closed" way. The inner master has caused the carriage to break down to force the coachman to stop. Illness comes at the end of a cycle of densification, when our resistance to change has crystalized and hardened. It is then necessary to repeat old patterns and experiences, reliving them in order to integrate them and change, if possible, the memories of one's holographic consciousness. This repetition can be done with a heightened awareness, and its success depends on the understanding we have of the origin of the illness and on our ability to decipher and accept the illness's message. Illness facilitates two things. First, it frees up tension that has been stored in us, and in this sense it plays an important role as a regulator. Illness also serves as a warning signal that is every bit as precise as trauma. It speaks to us very clearly about what is happening inside us and gives us revealing information for the future.

Inasmuch as it's a passive, yin message, illness is ultimately a flight, a weakening of the person experiencing it, and it is sometimes experienced unconsciously as a defeat of some sort. The carriage has broken down, and even if it has been repaired it is not as solid as a new carriage or at least doesn't inspire as much confidence in its owner. Consciously or not, illness represents an inability to understand, admit, or even simply feel the inner distortion that is the underlying cause of the illness. We don't know how to do things differently or, worse still, we think we haven't been strong enough to resist the illness. If we are able to draw a deeper lesson from the illness, after recovering we will develop inner immunity; otherwise we will weaken further and will tend to get sick more easily. The more long-lived the tension that needs to be cleared, the more serious the illness.

The difference between the passive/yin character of illness and the active/yang character of trauma is fundamental and is observable in the way in which the physical body resolves these two. In the case of trauma, the body repairs the damage through the miraculous phenomenon of healing. The healing is active because it is the traumatized cells or those of the same type that reconstitute themselves. The coachman himself can deal with it. In the case of illness, the body repairs itself using the immune system. This process is passive in the sense that the cells that intervene are of a different type from those that are sick. In this case you need to call in a mechanic to repair the carriage. The help, the assistance, the solution comes from the outside, from foreign elements (white blood cells for example), whereas in the case of trauma it is the traumatized part that helps itself, repairs itself, using its own cells.

The Freudian Slip

The Freudian slip, a concept that is part of classic psychoanalysis, refers to a "slip of the tongue" or an error in memory or physical action that reveals some unconscious aspect of the mind. In speaking of these missteps (called *parapraxes*), Freud gave us extraordinary insight into how an element of personal psychology interacts with the mind-body. He said that in our slipups, our clumsy and accidental speech and gestures, we are expressing or freeing up inner tension that we haven't been able or even known how to free up any other way. When we make such a blunder it expresses what in fact our real thoughts are.

What has always surprised me is that Freud used the term *slip* for these acts. When they are referred to in this way, they are automatically perceived as mistakes, as something that is not appropriate and should be avoided (at least by most individuals). That's a pity because it means we usually try to avoid these expressions by more effectively employing our inner censor. I prefer to call this kind of revealing expression a "score," even if the tangible result is not what the person's conscious self expected because this act is the real manifestation of an attempt by the nonconscious to communicate with the conscious. It's a message, sometimes coded, in which the nonconscious expresses an inner tension by telling the conscious that something doesn't make sense, something doesn't fit. The inner master is pulling on the reins held by the sleeping coachman, hoping that the shock produced by running over a hole or a bump is going to wake the driver up.

Like the physiological messages from the nonconscious that I spoke of earlier (in which category this kind of message also belongs) the successful act, the "score," can take one of three forms. It can be a matter of a slipup in language, that is, a mistake in verbal expression (using one word in place of another). It can be a clumsy gesture (spilling your glass of wine on someone or breaking an object that holds a certain value to the owner). Or it can involve a more traumatic act such as a cut or sprain or getting into a car accident. Freud spoke of these as "slips" because they *appear* to be mistakes, that is, negative. The reason is quite simple. Our nonconscious behaves like a child. When a child finds that her parents are not paying enough attention to her, not listening to her, she does what she needs to do to change that. If the child is an infant in a crib, she cries loudly and that works to bring her parents around. Later, she might try to do the same thing by breaking a plate, bringing bad marks home from school, or beating up her little brother. In the case of the Freudian slip we are like the parents who are too busy to realize what the needs of our inner child are. So we react only when the call becomes troublesome. Prior to the slipup we really didn't know what our nonconscious was trying to tell us.

It should also be noted that the nonconscious also sends us lots of positive messages, such as in dreams or the kind of messages I speak about in the following section on the mirror effect. But all too often we are not able or ready to hear messages from the nonconscious, and so the nonconscious, the inner master, moves on to the next stage, which is represented by the Freudian slip. These messages reveal a great deal if we are only willing to listen. If communication still flows between the conscious and the nonconscious—that is, if it has not been cut short by an overly dominant conscious—the message will come in the form of physical or psychological tension, nightmares, minor slips of the tongue, the breaking of meaningful objects, and so forth. If the communication between the two is of poor quality or almost nonexistent, the message will need to be stronger and louder (when the line is bad on the telephone, we sometimes have to shout to be heard by the other party). Thus the message will manifest as an accident or a conflict in order to provoke the kind of trauma I spoke about earlier. We can also manage to fall sick (catch a cold, drink or eat too much or not enough, etc.). And if communication is entirely cut off, that is when we develop a serious illness (autoimmune disease, cancer, etc.).

The Mirror Effect

Before going that far, life always offers us ways of getting information from our nonconscious and reflecting on it in relation to what is happening in our life. These messages are sent constantly by our environment and provide us with accurate and very substantive information to help us understand who we are and the meaning of our experiences. This is called the *mirror effect*. In fact, life speaks to us to offer guidance in numerous ways—we just need to listen. By observing what is happening around us and noticing who is in our environment, we have an inexhaustible field for understanding ourself. The mirror effect is an integral part of understanding life. As Carl Jung said, "In others we perceive the thousand facets of ourself."

So what is this mirror effect? For me, it has been one of the hardest philosophical concepts to fathom in my own personal journey. It means that everything we see in others and that forms part of others is nothing other than a reflection of ourself. When something pleases us in someone, generally it relates to a part of ourself that we don't dare believe in or that we don't dare express. Up to this point the principle is acceptable, but let's take it further. When we can't stand something in another person, it means that the trait is also a facet of ourself—something in that person is a part of us too and it's something we can't stand, so we refuse to see it, to accept it, and we cannot tolerate it in the other person because it is a reflection of something in ourself.

Just think about it honestly. What is the only part of your body that you can never see with your own eyes, even though you might be the greatest contortionist in the world? It's your face! Now what does this face represent, what is it for? It represents your identity, as in the photo that appears on your driver's license or passport. The only way you can see your own face is to look in a mirror. In it you see your reflection, the image that is sent back to you.

Similarly, in life the mirror is another person. What we see and what the mirror sends back to us is a faithful reflection of ourself, of what is happening within us. All this is even more striking if we absorb the fact that we actually choose the people we encounter. What a slap in the face that can be! What a blow when, for example, we often meet people who are unfair. That obliges us to reflect on our own unfair treatment of others. Let's ponder our own greed if we frequently meet greedy people, or our own infidelity if we are often betrayed.

Of course, as I've often done myself, we don't see, we don't find in ourself that which displeases us or bothers us in another person. But if we are completely honest, if we endeavor without judgment to really observe ourself, we will quickly discover just how the other person is like us and how we are like him or her. Life is designed so that we only see and are only attracted by what interests us, what concerns us. I was struck a few years ago when I decided one day to buy a particular car. It had been on the market for about a year. Starting from the time when I decided to buy it I constantly saw this car on the streets. There certainly weren't more of them than on any day prior to my decision, but my attention was specifically drawn by this particular model. In just the same way we see in the other person what interests us, what concerns us.

Another aspect of the mirror effect is that the nonconscious, our inner master, leads us to meet suitable people. This principle works in both a negative sense and in a positive sense. It is what determines how when we really want something, we will meet, as if by chance, people, books, or radio or television programs that are going to help us. This is what Jung terms *synchronicity.* Conversely, it is this same principle that has us meet inappropriate people or puts us in difficult situations when there is something we need to learn or understand, or to change our attitude about ourself and life. It is sometimes difficult to grasp or accept this, but in every case the question to ask is: "What do I have to learn from this situation?" or "What does this situation have to teach me?" If we ask this sincerely, the reply is quick to arrive. Tibetan Buddhist lamas say that in life our best teachers, those who get us moving ahead in life, are our worst enemies, those who make us suffer the most.

However, in many cases we can't hear the message represented by the negative person or situation, which is only trying to tell us what we need to work on or be aware of in life. If this is the case, the nonconscious will repeat the message in the form of slipups, traumas, or illness. All these things speak to us—we just have to learn how to decipher the language of the message. In the second part of this book we are going to do just that, by studying the different parts of the body and in particular, their functions. This might seem pointless because everybody is supposed to know what an arm, a leg, a stomach, or a lung is for, right? But we must understand that there is meaning attached to each part of the body outside of mere function, and this includes psychological projection. With such an understanding we can begin to extract meaning from the tensions and imbalances that manifest in one part of the body or another. If that is what you're most interested in, you can skip directly to the second part of the book.

But before we get to the specific manifestations of imbalance in particular parts of the body, it seems to me useful to explain how these manifestations happen and what they depend on. Based on the overall presentation of human reality, we have just seen *why* things operate in this way—the physical manifestations are cries for attention from the inner master to the conscious mind when we have strayed too far from our true Life Path. Now we are going to explore the mechanism by which these messages function in us. This is the domain of energy, of the energetic understanding of the human being. In chapters 2 and 3 I will be presenting the Taoist codification of the different types of energy and notably their structuring in the body. Yin, yang, acupuncture meridians, chakras—delving into these concepts will allow us to energetically connect together all of the parts of ourselves that modern science separates and divides up. In this way, we can once again assign meaning to the expression of each part—meaning that we have doubtless forgotten in our habit of looking at ourselves from a modern Western perspective.

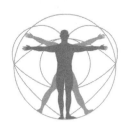

2

Between Heaven and Earth

The Human Being as a Microcosm of the Universe

It is not heaven that prematurely cuts life's thread in men; it is that men, by their mindless wandering, attract death to themselves in the middle of their lives.

MENCIUS

Among the world traditions that codify and preserve a holistic conceptualization of the human being, Taoism is for me the most profound. Taoist philosophy centers on the fundamental idea of "the all that is in everything." This means that the individual human being is a microcosm of the universe, the whole, all that is. As we shall see, this everything-in-everything principle as it is applied physiologically says that the human body is built according to the same rules as the entire cosmos, and therefore it must respect the same natural forces and cyclic laws.

Of course the most recognizable natural cycles are the seasons, the phases of the moon, and the cycle of day and night, but there are untold others. Humans, metaphysically positioned between Heaven and Earth according to Taoism, receive energy from each. Humans serve as catalyzers, transforming the cosmic energy of Heaven within, thus "humanizing" it and in so doing advancing their development. Implicit in this concept is the idea that human beings cannot be disconnected from the whole, from the all—each is intrinsic to the other, as confirmed by modern quantum physics, which confirms the everything-in-everything principle and posits string theory as the ultimate explanatory framework for understanding the universe. In fact, owing to the interconnectedness of everything, modern researchers verify that they themselves, along with their measuring instruments, influence the outcome of experiments. These results force us to question some of our most deeply held assumptions. Is reality not as segmented as a certain Cartesian view would have us believe!

Quantum physicists such as Wolfgang Pauli (1900–1958) and David Bohm (1917–1992) made great strides forward when they collaborated with figures from diverse fields such as analytical psychologist C. G. Jung (1875–1961) and philosopher and spiritual teacher J. Krishnamurti. More recently, "holistic physicist" F. David Peat works with Native Americans, in particular the Blackfoot people, because their particular way of describing and understanding the world is such that they do not speak about or describe things or objects, but rather processes and functions. Fritjof Capra shows clearly in his best-selling book *The Tao of Physics* how, through the quantum approach, he rediscovered all the laws described thousands of years ago by Taoist philosophers. (I want to remind the reader here that, contrary to what certain people might think, Taoism is a philosophy of life and not a religion.) In this chapter and the next we will see how these Taoist views help enrich the understanding of things and their interactions.

Lao-tzu and Confucius, the ancient theoretician-scribes of Taoist philosophy who elucidated Taoism's central premise of yin and yang, were philosophers and scholars, not religious figures. Using the conceptual axes of yin and yang, along with the law of the Five Elements (or *Five Principles,* a term I prefer), which are the five types of chi (life-force energy) dominating at different times, they codified and structured all life-forms in the universe, including human beings. They explored these principles through their empirical observation of things and by means of their ability to open themselves up to higher levels of consciousness.

Yin and Yang

All things exist and function on the basis of the permanent and immutable interaction of two forces, the yin and the yang. This yin/yang polarity is totally complementary. In fact, even though these two forces are opposed, they are never antagonistic or monolithic. At any given moment when one of the two reaches its zenith it always carries within itself the beginning or birthing point of the other force. Everything that exists is therefore constructed, observed, and understood around this concept. There is day; there is night. There is Heaven; there is Earth. There is black and white, high and low, young and old, beautiful and ugly, positive and negative, hot and cold, and so forth, ad infinitum. The polar yin/yang structuring of all materialization of life appears clearly, along with the understanding that nothing is totally one or the other, as is shown in the famous symbol of the Tao in which each part carries within it a point of the color of its opposite.

All planes of life are represented by the *bagua* of the I Ching, or Book of Changes, the classic Chinese text that expresses all the laws that

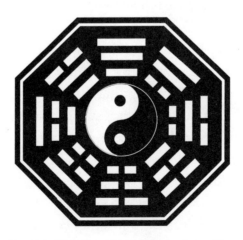

Fig. 2.1. The Tai Chi, symbol of the Tao

govern the universe. Specifically, the bagua are the broken or unbroken lines that represent all possible combinations of yin and yang depicted in trigrams. Each trigram, composed of three lines that are yin (broken) or yang (unbroken), corresponds to a representation of family life (father, mother, son, daughter, etc.) or nature (wind, thunder, marsh, mountain, etc.) and symbolizes all the potentialities through which life expresses itself. When two such trigrams are combined it makes a hexagram, of which there are sixty-four in the I Ching. Although often called a work of divination, the I Ching is more precisely a tool for conveying the inner messages and signs sent to us by our own inner master or inner guide. Later on we will see how important these messages are.

As we can see in the table below, all manifestations of life can be classified in relation to yin and yang. Of course it is impossible to list all life-forms, so I only offer a few examples here. What's essential is to grasp the *spirit* of these divisions.

YIN AND YANG

Yin	Yang
The moon, winter, water, north, cold, night, feminine, mother, the passive, the negative, receiving, feeling, affect, depths, black, dark, shadow, the inner, the hidden, space, the bottom, the right side, soft, flexible, the manifest, the tangible, gesture, the real, even (vs. odd), matter, quantity, substance, etc.	The sun, summer, fire, south, hot, day, masculine, father, the active, the positive, gift, action, reflecting, the surface, white, clear, light, the outer, appearance, time, top, left, hard, stiff, the unmanifest, the intangible, thought, virtual, odd (vs. even), energy, quality, essence, etc.

With their unwavering logic, Taoist philosophers applied this conceptualization of yin and yang to the whole universe, the macrocosm, as well as to the human being, the microcosm. In a human body, for example, the bottom is therefore yin and the top yang; the right is yin and the left is yang; the front is yin and back is yang; the depths are yin and the surface yang.

I must emphasize that the concepts of yin and yang are not static—in fact, quite the contrary. They are completely relative to the level of observation and to the point observed. If the cold is yin, the less cold of the cold is yang and the coldest of the cold is yin. If the dark is yin, the less dark is yang, and the most dark is yin. If the hot is yang, the less hot is yin and the most hot is yang. If the bright is yang, the less bright is yin and the most bright is yang. That is to say the yin is always the yin of something, and the yang is always the yang of something. Each one takes its meaning *in relation to its complement,* in the same way that there is a right hand because there is a left hand, or there is a top because there is a bottom, and so forth.

The Five Principles

The second conceptual basis of Taoism is the law of the Five Principles, often called the Five Elements, and also known as the Five Phases, Five Agents, Five Movements, and Five Processes. I prefer the term *Five Principles* because they are the existential basis of the entire universe that contains all elements. Empirical observation led the ancient Chinese sages to realize that the Five Principles manage, structure, and represent everything that exists in the universe. These Five Principles are Metal, Earth, Fire, Water, and Wood.

The Five Principles are in continual interaction according to two laws that are both extremely simple and extremely precise: addition and subtraction. These two laws define and manage relationships among the Five Principles; they were established and codified based on observation of the natural laws. The ancient Taoist sages noticed that in our universe all interrelationships are managed by addition and subtraction (multiplication being only a summing up of additions and division a summing up of subtractions). We can then either add something or subtract something (take it away). They extracted two laws from these factors, the only two laws that manage interactions among the Five Principles.

We don't really know the origin of the law of Five Principles. It is lost in antiquity and was forged over time, little by little, from in-depth observation of all the cycles of nature such as climatic, seasonal, energetic, botanical, and other cycles. This observation led Taoists to con-

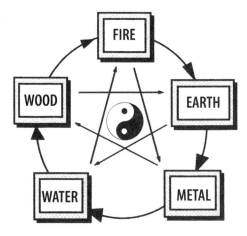

Fig. 2.2. The Five Principles

clude that the universe is subject to systematic cyclic functioning. This cyclic functioning operates continually according to two simultaneous cycles: a *creation cycle* and a *control cycle*. These two cycles govern the interdependent relationships among the Five Principles, which are the existential basis of the universe. In this law of the Five Principles we find all the elements that we already know about the Tao, since each principle has a form that is more fully or less fully yin or yang.

There is complete symbolism associated with each of the Five Principles, making it possible to determine the whole, complex extent of what each represents. Each of the elements that constitute the Five Principles corresponds to a specific planet, cardinal direction, season, climate, color, taste, scent, type of food, and human organ. Each is associated with a yin meridian and a yang meridian, a time of day, a psychological type, a morphological type, and so forth. This rich symbolism shows us the fundamental importance of this energetic law, which is the basis of the Taoist understanding of human beings and also applies to all other manifestations of life.*

---

*For more information on this subject, please refer to my book *L'Harmonie des énergies* (The Harmony of Energies).

The four seasons of the year, for example, can be transposed to other cycles in life. For example, they fit perfectly into the delineation of a day, morning being the spring, midday being summer, afternoon being autumn, and night being winter. They can be applied to the life of a person as well, birth and early childhood being spring, youth (up to age forty) being summer, maturity (up to the sixties) being autumn, and old age and death being winter. This seasonal division can in fact be overlaid on any designation of time, such as a project, an illness, the building of a house, or the digestion of a meal. Everything is in everything.

The Five Principles are governed by the law of creation and the law of control. The law of creation is derived from the operation of addition and for this reason is sometimes called the "Mother-Son law." With a flawless logic it defines the first form of relationship among the Five Principles: Wood generates Fire, which generates Earth, which generates Metal, which generates Water, which generates Wood, which in its turn generates Fire, and so forth. Let's look at this further. Wood is what nourishes, feeds, and produces Fire. Therefore, that is what creates it. It is also logical to say the Fire nourishes and feeds Earth. Farmers set fire to a stubble field to fertilize the earth with ash. Just as logical is the idea that Earth produces or creates Metal (metal ore is extracted from the earth). It can seem less obvious that Metal creates Water, but it is good to remember that oxidizing metal frees up hydrogen molecules needed by water. Let's remember that water is needed for oxidation, and also that when we want to produce water using catalysis based on oxygen and hydrogen, a metallic electrode is needed. Finally, when metal is heated it becomes liquid. This last explanation takes into consideration the other side of the relationship by considering that Water is the "son" of Metal. The child in his mother's belly nourishes himself from her, "eats" her. He "consumes" her just as water "eats" metal since it corrodes it. And finally, it is fairly obvious that Water generates Wood, since all plants need to be irrigated to be able to grow.

The second law, that of control, derives from the operation of subtraction. This law defines a second form of relationship among the Five

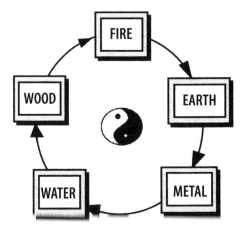

Fig. 2.3. The law of creation

Principles that is similarly explicit. Wood controls Earth, Fire controls Metal, Earth controls Water, Metal controls Wood, and Water controls Fire. Here too the explication is simple and logical. Wood controls Earth, that is, it masters it. We can also say that it inhibits it. This is why to stabilize the dunes or prevent the erosion of soil we plant vegetation. It is also clear that Fire controls Metal. The blacksmith uses fire to forge, melt, and work metal by giving it a form. That Earth controls Water is clear by observing a flowing spring. Earth absorbs water, and

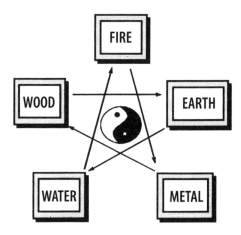

Fig. 2.4. The law of control

we use it to seal off ponds or contain rivers and streams. It is equally clear that Metal controls Wood; after all, we cut and fashion a piece of wood with a metal tool. That Water controls Fire is pretty obvious, since we've all experienced extinguishing the one with the other.

So these are the two simple, natural laws that define the interdependence among the Five Principles. The two laws position and specify the reciprocal influences (and their relative importance), and consequently the importance of all the intervening criteria that are related to them (season, time of day, imbalance, form, mind, individual typology, etc.). They also identify the specific quality of energy that circulates in our meridians. The table below provides the correspondence between each of the Five Principles and some of the elements to which they are related. Since everything is in everything, we can say that each of the Five Principles is based on these two laws and five subprinciples. In Metal, for example, we have once again Earth, Water, Wood, Fire, and of course Metal, which constitute this principle. The everything-in-everything principle is illustrated by the idea of a hall of mirrors. In the famous one at the palace of Versailles, when you position yourself before a mirror, because of the presence of other mirrors behind you, the image reflected to you is your own but you see a practically infinite number of mirrors getting smaller and smaller following one another that also contain your image.

Principle	Wood	Fire	Earth	Metal	Water
Cardinal direction	East	South	Center	West	North
Seasonal energy	Spring	Summer	End of season	Autumn	Winter
Climatic energy	Wind	Heat	Humidity	Dryness	Cold
Daily energy	Morning	Midday	Afternoon	Evening	Night
Energy of color	Green	Red	Yellow	White	Black
Food tastes	Acid, sour	Bitter	Sweet	Spicy	Salty

Principle	Wood	Fire	Earth	Metal	Water
Strong life-force moments	Birth	Youth	Maturity	Old age	Death
Major organ	Liver	Heart	Spleen/pancreas	Lungs	Kidneys
Viscus	Gallbladder	Small intestine	Stomach	Large intestine	Urinary bladder
General physiology	Eye, muscles	Tongue, blood vessels	Flesh, connective tissue	Skin, nose, hair	Bone, marrow, ears
Sense organs	Sight	Touch	Taste	Smell	Hearing
Types of secretions	Tears	Sweat	Saliva	Mucus	Urine
Physiological symptomatology	Nails	Complexion	Lips	Body hair	Head of hair
Typology of mind	Perception, imagination, creation	Intelligence, passion, consciousness	Thought, memory, reason, realism	Intention, rigor, action/things	Severity, fertile will, decision
Energetic typology	Mobilization, exteriorization	Expansion	Distribution	Interiorization	Concentration
Psychology/ passions	Susceptibility, anger	Joy, pleasure, violence	Reflecting, worries	Sadness, grief, concern	Anxiety, fear
Psychology/ virtues	Harmony	Brilliance, ostentation	Circumspection, penetration	Clarity, integrity, purity	Rigor, severity
Psychology/ qualities	Elegance, Beauty	Prosperity	Abundance	Firmness, sense of accomplishment	Sense of listening
Numbers in Chinese astrology	3 and 8	2 and 7	0 and 5	4 and 9	1 and 6
Associated planet	Jupiter	Mars	Saturn	Venus	Mercury

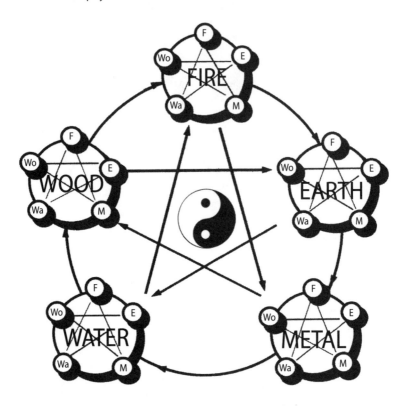

Fig. 2.5. Everything is in everything.

Thus, like the hall of mirrors analogy, the Taoist concept of everything-in-everything concludes that each of the Five Principles is found to be itself composed of five similar subprinciples, which, in turn are composed of sub-subprinciples, and so forth. All this also looks very much like what mathematician Benoit Mandelbrot (1924–2010) rediscovered and called *fractals*.

How Energies Function to Achieve Structure and Balance in the Body

The word *Tao* translates as "path," "method," "principle," or "way." Taoist philosophy is based on the idea that there is a central organizing principle of the universe, a natural order or a "way of Heaven," the

Tao, that one can come to know by living in harmony with nature (the Earth) and hence with the cosmos and the universe. According to Taoist cosmology, the appearance of human beings took place as a result of two things: the action of the Original Principle, the person's Shen before birth, his or her individual essence of life (which can also be called the *divine principle, primordial energy, cosmic consciousness,* depending on your personal beliefs and cultural traditions), and the interaction of Heaven and Earth as a manifestation of the interplay between yang and yin. These two energetic forces, yang and yin, have a point of meeting, convergence, and transformation: the human being.

As a point of meeting and transformation between the yang energy of Heaven and the yin energy of Earth, the individual person combines these two energies within himself or herself to form what we call *essential energy,* which is something like the raw fuel used to power a car. This fuel in turn is combined with another energy called *ancestral energy,* which is something like an additive used to supplement the fuel we use to run the car. The resulting amalgam gives rise to a new form of energy that I call *life-force energy,* which is to say our personal premium-grade gasoline. This life-force energy is an integral part of each one of us and allows us to exist in time as a singular, unique being. In such a way each one of us has certain strengths and weaknesses, good qualities and faults, excesses and deficiencies.

Throughout the course of life we receive and integrate the energy of Heaven (through the breath) and the energy of the Earth (as nutrition finds its way into the stomach). The way in which we consume both forms of energy and then assimilate them, combining them to form essential energy, determines the quality and texture of that energy, which is our raw fuel. Then the combination of essential energy with ancestral energy (more about this follows) determines the quality of our premium fuel. Premium fuel involves our strength at each moment—our resistance, our typology of character, and the quality of energy we transmit (especially if we procreate). Thus ancestral energy—the fuel additive—plays an important role as a qualitative and quantitative

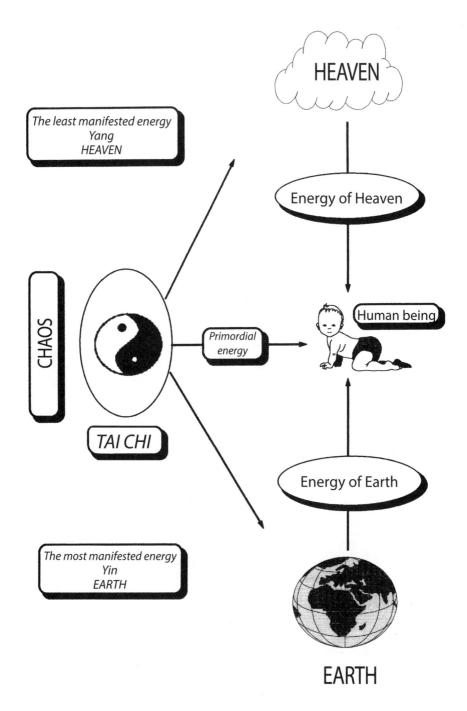

Fig. 2.6. The human being between Heaven and Earth

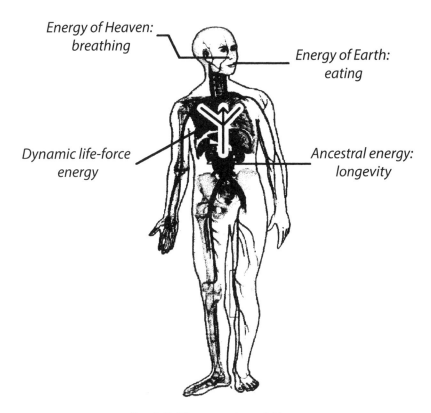

Fig. 2.7. The energies within us

regulator of life-force energy. In fact, if the quality of one's essential energy leaves something to be desired because it shows an imbalance (too much energy of Heaven or of Earth, or possibly a poor quality of those energies), the ancestral energy will intervene and play its regulating role by drawing on its "stock" in order to reestablish the qualitative and quantitative balance that has been disturbed.

The way we assimilate each of these forms of energy, plus their quality and influence, can be predetermined if we do not bring our attention to them or if we do not do a good job of working on each form of energy. We need to know them and want to see them evolve. Intelligent nutrition, that is, well-balanced and sufficient; a physical exercise regimen that involves the breath; plus an appropriate behavioral and psychological attitude can help us obtain an essential energy of satisfactory quality.

Let's return for a moment to that special "additive" we call ancestral energy, which plays a determining role for each of us. As its name indicates, ancestral energy carries ancestral memories. It is the memory of Shen and the human being, thus it is the root of both. It is through that energy that each person is connected to the whole of humanity and to humanity's history from the very beginning. We could think of it by using the image of water coming from a spring high on a mountain. Even though it is running now in the present moment, the water carries the whole history of the mountain, with all the minerals and substances coming from the mountain itself and also from its glaciers, which formed eons ago. Thus the snow that melts into water today may have fallen thousands of years ago. Similarly, through ancestral energy we are permanently connected to our entire history (i.e., to our Akashic Records) as well as to the history of our family lineage (i.e., our ancestors). In a way this ancestral energy brings us into contact with the collective unconscious and the Jungian archetypes.

The quantity of ancestral energy varies from one person to the next and is set once for each person at the time of conception. It diminishes during the course of one's life according to a given biological rhythm, like a reservoir that gradually empties with a tap that cannot be closed completely. The biological rhythm will speed up or slow down in response to the demands placed upon it by our behavior, in other words, according to the management of this resource. Ancestral energy determines longevity for each one of us. We can easily understand how our attitudes toward eating and toward physical and mental self-care act not only in the moment in terms of one's health, but also over time in terms of one's longevity and vitality. We need to remember that it is this ancestral energy that compensates for all cases of imbalance.*

---

*Note that modern medicine can keep a body "alive" in a vegetative state even after it has used up all of its ancestral energy, but in the normal state of affairs consciousness leaves the body and the physical body dies when all of its ancestral energy has been depleted.

Now let us return to the subject of life-force energy. As we have stated, it is made up of essential energy and ancestral energy. This deep alchemy takes place inside each one of us at a very specific location: between the two kidneys. Taoists symbolize it with the image of a little three-legged pot. This energetic center corresponds to the deep well from which the life force springs forth in us. Yin and yang, along with the Five Principles, regulate and govern this life-force energy. It spreads throughout the whole body, nourishing it and defending it based on the yin/yang dynamic.

The life-force energy circulates in energetic circuits called *meridians*. It plays its part while respecting interactions that are defined by the Five Principles and according to the polarities of that law. Starting from this three-legged pot, the life-force energy begins its circulation. It moves up the central channel, which is the channel of the "Kundalini" or "Chong Mai" (vital energy). It then gets distributed throughout the whole body and the organs through smaller and more specific channels—the famous meridians of acupuncture, which Taoists think of as streams or rivers that irrigate the whole organism. A part of this energy circulates on the surface of the body or the organs to defend them while another part enters more deeply to nourish them.

How Energies Move in the Body: The Meridians

There are twelve meridians in the body that are related to specific organs and are either yin or yang, along with an additional two complementary meridians that have to do with the front of the body for yin energy and the back of the body for yang energy—the Functional Channel (or Conception Vessel) on the front of the body and the Governor Channel (or Governing Vessel) on the back of the body. Below you will find the names of the twelve basic meridians and the organs associated with them.

	Yin	Yang
Organ meridian	Lung	Large Intestine
	Spleen/Pancreas	Stomach
	Heart	Small Intestine
	Kidney	Urinary Bladder
	Heart Protector/Pericardium	Triple Heater
	Liver	Gall Bladder

Our "premium gas" flows throughout our body, both deeply and on the surface, following these very precisely defined pathways. Although the meridians are energetic pathways and as such do not correspond to any specific physiological circuit, they do exist (as confirmed by modern science), and they support the functioning of our entire human reality—physical, psychological, and spiritual. Even though the meridians are assigned the names of the specific organs they affect, the meridians do not only play a physiological role; they have a very important psychological role as well. In fact, they connect the body and the mind inasmuch as the energy they convey serves equally to support the functioning of the organ as well as the psychology associated with that organ. Based on the meridians, we are able to make connections between things within us.

The circulation of energy, or chi, takes place unchangeably according to a well-defined spatial and temporal circuit. Starting from the central channel it unfolds according to a precise daily cycle. From the Lung meridian it moves to the Large Intestine meridian, then to the Stomach meridian. From there it travels to the Spleen/Pancreas meridian, and from there it goes to the Heart meridian, then to the Small Intestine meridian, to the Urinary Bladder meridian, and from there to the Kidney meridian. It continues through the Heart Protector meridian (also called the Pericardium meridian), then to the Triple Heater meridian, to the Gall Bladder meridian, and finally to the Liver meridian. After that the cycle begins anew and continues in this same way throughout a twenty-four-hour period, each stage lasting two hours.

The circulation of life-force energy produces during its cycle what are called "energetic tides," periods of force and preponderant circulation of this energy in each meridian that last for about two hours each. These represent the strong energetic periods for each meridian and for each organ or viscus associated with that meridian. On the other hand, they do not correspond to nor do they define the energetic relationships and interactions among the meridians that we will come to later on, which are defined by the Five Principles.

All this helps us understand a bit better the Taoist conception of the flow of energy, which is what the science of chronobiology—a field of biology that examines periodic (cyclic) phenomena in living organisms—is in the process of rediscovering today. We are not solid mechanisms but very much the opposite. Each period and hour of the day corresponds to times of strength or vulnerability for each of our organs as well as for the psychology that is associated with each of them.

The twelve organ-related meridians and the two complementary meridians circulate energy throughout the entire body. Each one of the organ meridians passes through identical spots on the two sides of the body, right and left, following a different path for each meridian. Following the logic of what we covered earlier concerning laterality, the energy will have a yin meaning when referring to the right side and a yang meaning when referring to the left side. Finally, each meridian is itself of a yin or a yang nature and is associated with an organ when it is yin and with a viscus when it is yang.

It would be good at this point to clarify the concepts of organ and viscera in the Chinese energetic codification. *Viscus* is a term for any organ inside of the body. *Viscera,* the plural of *viscus,* is a term used to describe all the organs inside the cavities of the body; however, *viscera* more commonly refers to all of the organs inside of the abdomen. Viscera inside the abdominal area are sometimes referred to as *guts* or *innards.* Each season has both an organ and a viscus associated with it that represents the yin and yang polarities manifested in the physical body. In traditional Chinese medicine, *organ* is the term used for yin organs and

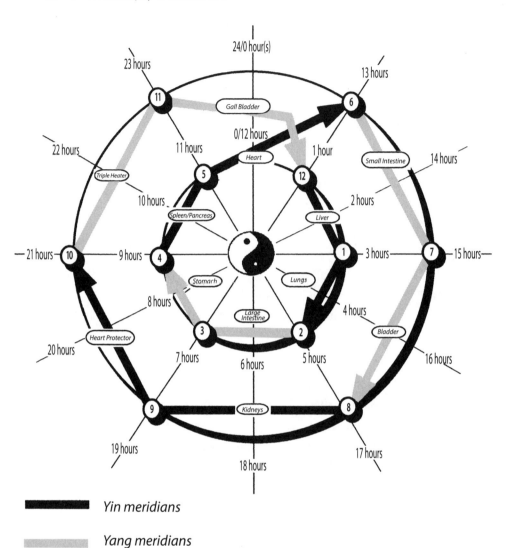

Yin meridians

Yang meridians

Fig. 2.8. The cycles of the circulation of life-force energy
according to solar time*

*Translator's note: Solar time is recorded according to the twenty-four-hour clock on
the lines that radiate beyond the big circles. Midnight, or 24:00, hours is at the top of
the biggest circle, and noon, or 12:00 hours, is at the top of the inner of the two big
circles. Note that the meridian lines move in two-hour stretches and begin at 3 a.m. At
3 a.m. you see the number 1 as the first two-hour cycle of the twelve two-hour periods
of the "meridian clock."

viscera is the term used for yang organs. They are: heart, spleen/pancreas, lungs, kidneys, and liver for the organs, and small intestine, stomach, large intestine, urinary bladder, and gallbladder for the viscera.

Lungs	Yin	03:00 to 05:00 solar time (3 a.m. to 5 a.m.)
Large intestine	Yang	05:00 to 07:00 solar time (5 a.m. to 7 a.m.)
Stomach	Yang	07:00 to 09:00 solar time (7 a.m. to 9 a.m.)
Spleen/pancreas	Yin	09:00 to 11:00 solar time (9 a.m. to 11 a.m.)
Heart	Yin	11:00 to 13:00 solar time (11 a.m. to 1 p.m.)
Small intestine	Yang	13:00 to 15:00 solar time (1 p.m. to 3 p.m.)
Urinary bladder	Yang	15:00 to 17:00 solar time (3 p.m. to 5 p.m.)
Kidneys	Yin	17:00 to 19:00 solar time (5 p.m. to 7 p.m.)
Heart Protector	Yin	19:00 to 21:00 solar time (7 p.m. to 9 p.m.)
Triple Heater	Yang	21:00 to 23:00 solar time (9 p.m. to 11 p.m.)
Gallbladder	Yang	23:00 to 01:00 solar time (11 p.m. to 1 a.m.)
Liver	Yin	01:00 to 03:00 solar time (1 a.m. to 3 a.m.)

What is particularly fascinating to me about the deep logic of Taoist philosophy is the way in which the ancient sages determined which organs and viscera are yin and which are yang. We are told this, in fact, as an amusing anecdote about the way in which the Taoists determined the yin or yang nature of the organs and viscera. But how "true" it is! As we have seen before, what is heavy and full corresponds to yin, and what is light and empty corresponds to yang. The Taoists, pragmatic and logical, took a container of water and immersed into this container, one after the other, each of the organs and viscera of an animal or human cadaver. Whatever floated (therefore being lighter than water) could only be yang in nature, which is the case of each viscus, and whatever sank (therefore being heavier than water) could only be yin in nature, which is the case of all the organs. I often use this connection to water and its density to explain yin, yang, and the Tao (or rather Tai Chi, which is the manifestation or expression of the Tao). Yin is the most manifested form of things, while yang is the least manifested form of things. Tai Chi is the synergy of the two. This can be understood from the example of water. Water is life and the source of life. It is the Tai Chi and the Tao. Its densest, most manifested form (therefore yin) is ice, and its most diffuse, least manifested form (therefore yang) is water vapor.

The final clarification that I want to bring to this discussion concerns the interactions among the meridians. These interactions are defined by the law of the Five Principles, each meridian being in direct relationship with one of these principles as indicated in the table below.

Meridian/Organ	Associated Principle
Lung	Metal yin
Large Intestine	Metal yang
Stomach	Earth yang
Spleen/Pancreas	Earth yin
Heart	Fire yin
Small Intestine	Fire yang
Urinary Bladder	Water yang
Kidney	Water yin
Heart Protector	Fire yin
Triple Heater	Fire yang
Gall Bladder	Wood yang
Liver	Wood yin

The Distribution of Yin and Yang in the Body

Upper and Lower

Let's return to the human body. As noted earlier, in the Taoist codification that which is below is yin and that which is above is yang. When

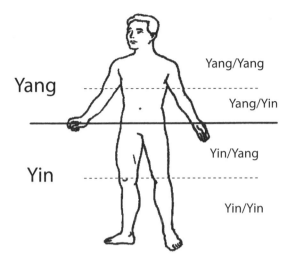

Fig. 2.9. Yin and yang distribution
in the upper and lower body

we relate that to the scale of the human body, the top of the body is then yang and the bottom is yin. We need to remember, though, the relativity of these concepts. If we observe the lower part of the body, which in relation to the whole body is yin, in the case of the leg the upper part will be yang and the lower part yin. It is exactly the same for the upper body, which is yang in relation to the whole body, but relatively speaking the upper part is yang and the lower part is yin. This relativity applies to the whole body. We are always going to be observing things starting from the macrocosm (what is biggest), and then refining toward the microcosm (what is smallest).

Let's take a simple example to illustrate this principle. A person is suffering from a knee problem. The knee is part of the leg, so the first level of relationship is with this person's yin since the legs are in the lower part of the body. But within the leg the knee is right in the middle, that is, right between yang and yin. It forms the meeting point, the joint between these two parts. Therefore, the second level of relationship is located between yang and yin. So it is in the relationship between the yang of the yin and the yin of the yin that the problem is to be found, and it is in that direction that we will be searching for the message and the eventual solution. We will be picking up this example again and refining the analysis further, specifically by elaborating on the meaning of yin and yang, but also by explaining the meaning of laterality in the role played by each part of the body.

Right and Left

We have also seen that yin and yang are related to laterality. Right is yin by nature, while left is yang. Objectively then, the right side of the body is related to yin while the left side is related to yang. However, once again we must apply the principle of relativity. The upper part of the body is yang and the lower part is yin. The left side of the body is yang and the right yin. The lower left is therefore yang within the yin zone; it is the yang of the yin. As for the lower right, it is yin within the yin zone. The upper part of the body is yang but the right is yin. This upper

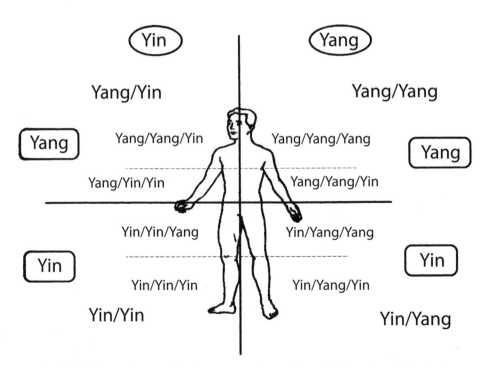

Fig. 2.10. Yin and yang distribution on the right and left sides of the body

right part is then yin within the yang part; it is the yin of the yang. The upper left, which is yang, is then the yang of the yang.

Let's come back to our example of someone suffering from a knee problem. We have already seen that it has to do with a problem in the yin part of the body concerning the joint or meeting point between yin and yang in this part of the body. If it has to do with the left knee, the laterality of which is yang, we can be more precise in saying that the problem is related to the yang dynamic of the person, to the yang part of his life. If it has to do with the right knee, since this side is yin, the person then has a problem with the yin dynamic, with the yin side of life. We can see how things are now becoming a little clearer.

Deep and Superficial

Earlier we saw that yin corresponds to the depths, to what is hidden, while yang is associated with what is on the surface, what is apparent. What is deep inside our body is, because of that, yin in nature—for example, the organs. What is on the surface—for example, the skin—is yang in nature. But here let's once again apply the principle of relativity. For what is deep and yin in nature, its surface will be yang and its depths will be yin. If we have, for example, a pulmonary infection, it will be the yin of this yin part of the body that will be involved. If, on the other hand, it concerns the pleura (the exterior envelope, the exterior surface of the lungs), it is then the yang of this yin part that is involved.

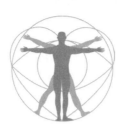

3

Connections
within the Body

The Five Principles and
the Twelve Organ Meridians

"My heart is afraid of suffering," said the young man to the alchemist one night as they were watching the moonless sky. "Tell your heart that fear of suffering is worse than suffering itself. And that no heart has ever suffered when it was in pursuit of its dreams."

PAULO COELHO, *THE ALCHEMIST*

Let us now take a look at how the parts of our body (organs and limbs) are not only interrelated, but how they are intrinsically connected to our psychological and spiritual dimensions. Here the Taoist conceptualization of interrelatedness overturns the Cartesian philosophy of dualism that dominates in the West and that separates the body-mind-spirit.

The connections between all the parts of the body and the connections to the external world are reflected in the meridians as grouped according to the Five Principles and as delineated by the principles (or elements) Metal, Earth, Fire, Water, and Wood. These connections also affect us on more subtle levels—on the psychological level, in our many reactions and attitudes, as well as on the mental and spiritual levels. All these connections are facilitated by chi, the life-force energy that circulates in the meridians according to the correspondences established by each of the Five Principles.

Therefore we are going first of all to approach the study of the twelve meridians of the human body following the guiding thread that interests us and proceeding principle by principle. This will allow us to be able to refer to the summary tables on the preceding pages.

Metal

Lung and Large Intestine Meridians

Metal governs everything that concerns our connection to the external world. Our ability to protect ourself when confronted by that world and how we handle external aggression both depend on the Metal principle. It is therefore our armor, our personal coat of mail. Its level of protection is instinctive, operates reflexively, and does not involve any kind of premeditated thought. It can make us reactive, even primal. Our level of perception is that of physical sensations. In a corresponding way, it also manages our ability to get rid of or expel aggression quickly.

Metal concerns our ability to cut through (as with a sword), to choose. It has to do with judiciousness, decision-making based on looking into the rightness of a situation. Hard choices, necessary choices that require being clear-cut, require Metal. Sometimes we need to stop functioning on the level of thoughtful reasoning (Earth) alone, which can rigidify when it becomes excessive. In such cases we have to depend on the element Metal in order to choose, to cut through. This is in the territory of intentionality, of will, referring to what is done forcefully, like a blade that cuts through things because it is harder than what it is cutting or what it is penetrating.

Two meridians are associated with the Metal principle—the Lung meridian and the Large Intestine meridian.

The Lung Meridian

The Lung meridian is associated with the Chinese astrological sign of the Tiger and the season of autumn. Its body pathway ends at the tip of the thumb of each hand, and it permits the absorption of chi on which life-force activity depends. This energy comes from external sources, notably in the form of oxygen (but not only that), and is transformed inside the human body into essential energy and then into life-force energy. Its role is to give strength and the ability to resist aggression coming from the outside world.

The Lung meridian manages the balance between the outside and the inside. It protects against the outside world (in the form of skin). It also works with physical energy and assists the heart in controlling energy coming from the air. This latter energy, associated with the blood, feeds the organs and the viscera. In addition, the Lung meridian participates actively in the quality of physical energy thanks to the transformations that it directs. In fact, to be able to correctly circulate through and feed the whole body, the energy of Earth (food) must combine with the energy of Heaven (air) to form essential energy. It seems clear that if this combining is not well-managed, the organism will not be well-nourished.

On the physiological level, this meridian corresponds to the breathing apparatus, including the skin, the nose, and the system of body hair. It is the Lung meridian that regulates the thermal balance of these areas and allows them to protect themselves, notably from climatic and environmental aggression. At the psychological level it is associated with the ability for self-defense when confronted by the world outside. It is associated with rigor, with acting on things, but also with interiorization in the sense of nonmanifestation and camouflage (armor). This can also be a form of intentionality, or intentional will. The predominant solar time slot of the Lung meridian is from 03:00 to 05:00 solar time (3 a.m. to 5 a.m.).

The Large Intestine Meridian

The Large Intestine meridian is associated with the Chinese astrological sign of the Hare and complements the Lung meridian. Like the Lung meridian it too is associated with autumn. It begins its path at the tip of each index finger, and its function is to transport and clear waste, thus it prevents the stagnation of chi. Because of this it influences excretion of organic solids (whereas the Urinary Bladder meridian plays the same role for organic liquids). The Large Intestine meridian clears what we have eaten (ingested) but not assimilated (accepted). It plays this role not only for food, however, but for everything connected to our psychological experiences. If the Large Intestine meridian is not working as it should, there will be difficulties with clearing in the whole body (in the lungs, intestines, kidneys, and urinary bladder) as well as in the psychology of the person. The Large Intestine meridian and the Lung meridian are complementary and are associated with the same physical and psychological areas. The predominant solar time slot of the Large Intestine meridian is between 05:00 and 07:00 (5 a.m. to 7 a.m.).

Earth

Stomach and Spleen/Pancreas Meridians

Earth energy is in charge of thought, contemplation, and meditation. Everything that involves memory, or more precisely with what has been experienced, depends on it. Reason, realism, and common sense are managed by the element Earth—as are worries and obsessive thinking. Earth energy is assimilated based on two meridians associated with this principle, the Stomach meridian and the Spleen/Pancreas meridian.

The Earth principle is in charge of our connection to matter in the sense of its mastery—owning it, dominating it, appropriating it, and exerting power over it. Earth allows us to digest and assimilate everything having to do with the tangible, material world. As with the other elements, this can run in both directions, so that jealousy and desire, but also abundance and prodigality all come from Earth. The meridians associated with the Earth principle are the Stomach meridian and the Spleen/Pancreas meridian.

The Stomach Meridian

The Stomach meridian, which is associated with the Chinese astrological sign of the Dragon and the "end of season," receives and transforms Earth energy through digestion.* Its body pathway ends at the tip of the second toe (the "foot's index finger"). This meridian regulates the stomach and the whole digestive tract and as such is in charge of digesting things both on the physiological plane (what we have eaten) as well as on the psychological plane (what we have assimilated in the form of events, experiences, etc.). It takes care of the reception of physical edibles (foodstuffs) and psychological edibles (events), including their temporary storage and transformation. It looks after everything that involves material reality, allowing us to master, possess, and appropriate the matter that we ingest.

The Stomach meridian is related to the movement of the limbs and the heat produced by the body, because the limbs help the stomach and the digestive tract operate properly. This meridian, which is connected to appetite, is also in charge of maternal milk production (the nourishment of someone else), the functioning of the genital glands, the ovaries, and menstruation. We can see how its connection to food is important because it manages what we receive (food as well as information) and also what we give (mother's milk) or what we transmit (education, training).

At a physiological level this meridian corresponds to the flesh, to the connective tissue, and to muscle mass (as does its complementary Spleen/Pancreas meridian). It is located physically at the mouth and lips. On the psychological plane it is associated with thought, memory, reason, and realism, as well as contemplation and worry. The Stomach meridian's predominant solar time slot is from 07:00 to 09:00 (7 a.m. to 9 a.m.).

---

*The "season" attributed to the Earth principle is a symbolic season that corresponds to the last eighteen days of each of the other seasons. For example, in the Chinese solar calendar the last 18 days of spring correspond to April 12 to April 30 and the last eighteen days of summer correspond to July 13 to July 31 and so forth.

The Spleen/Pancreas Meridian

The Spleen/Pancreas meridian is associated with the Chinese astrological sign of the Snake and, like the Stomach, corresponds to the "end of season." Its body pathway begins at the tip of the big toe on the inside of the foot. It is concerned with the glands of the digestive system, which are found in the mouth, the stomach, the gallbladder, and the small intestine, as well as with the mammary glands and the ovaries. It plays a pivotal role in the continuous distribution of food to the body. Food is not able to be assimilated directly by the organism and so its transformation into a form that can be assimilated is assured by the stomach and spleen/pancreas. This energy obtained from food is associated with the energy of the air thanks to the lungs, and is transformed into essential energy.

The digestive juices of the stomach are controlled by the spleen/pancreas, which makes an initial distinction between food it can use and the food it can't use. It also directs the transformation of absorbed liquids into usable form. In this way it regulates the ensemble of nutrition and energy in the body. The Spleen/Pancreas meridian is responsible for the type and quality of our relationship to the matter that we appropriate though digestion. This applies also to concerns about the material world and the possessiveness, insecurity, and anxiety connected to this world.

The spleen/pancreas's role in the management and regulation of sugars is fundamental. (In part 2 we will see how this allows us to understand diabetes in a different way than the allopathic medical model does.) On the physiological and psychological levels this meridian corresponds to the same element as the Stomach meridian. The predominant solar time for the Spleen/Pancreas meridian is from 09:00 to 11:00 (9 a.m. to 11 a.m.)

Fire

Heart, Small Intestine, Heart Protector, and Triple Heater Meridians

The Fire principle has to do with flames, with what burns in us. The flame is inner and relates to passion but also to the "luminous" aspect of a person, that is, to one's psychological and intellectual clarity. Brilliance, intelligence, mental acuity, and spirituality all depend on Fire. Seeing things clearly, free thinking, the power of understanding, and lightning-fast analysis belong to Fire. Consequently, Fire provides lucidity, but also its opposite, subjectivity.

The understanding we have of the world depends on the quality of our Fire. From Fire comes pleasure, joy, happiness, and satisfaction. The world of emotions depends on Fire, and the passion that it carries can sometimes become violent if it is excessive. Fire is the principle of high-flying expression, be it emotional, lyrical, or some other form. Optimism, enthusiasm, and a facility for elocution and expression depend on it, as does ardor, spiritedness, and one's willingness to help.

Two pairs of meridians are associated with the Fire principle: the Heart and Small Intestine meridians and the Heart Protector and Triple Heater meridians.

The Heart Meridian

The heart is associated with the Chinese astrological sign of the Horse and with summer. The Heart meridian begins in the armpit and runs down the inner arm, with its body pathway ending on the outside face of the tip of each little finger. It helps us adapt external stimulation to the internal condition of the individual body. Because of this it is intimately connected to emotional states, and it also regularizes the functioning of the whole body through its action on the brain and the five senses.

Taoists consider the heart to be the "emperor" of the organism and of the psyche. Intelligence and awareness depend on the heart. As we shall see, there is a very close connection between the heart, the Heart Protector meridian, and the brain. Any imbalance in the heart has repercussions on all the other meridians. It controls the distribution of blood and manages the vascular system. Since it is related to the tongue it also makes the distinguishing of tastes possible. On the physiological level the Heart meridian corresponds to the tongue and the blood vessels. Its presence is reflected in the complexion. On the psychological level this meridian is associated with awareness, intelligence, passion, and brilliance, but also with violence. It is love, but passionate love, love that burns and consumes. Its predominant solar time is between 11:00 and 13:00 (11 a.m. and 1 p.m.).

The Small Intestine Meridian

The Small Intestine meridian complements the Heart meridian and like the latter is also connected to the season of summer. Its body pathway begins at the tip of the little finger on each hand, and its Chinese astrology symbol is the Goat. The small intestine acts as a kind of personal advisor to the "emperor," the heart, which it assists by ensuring the assimilation of food by controlling the separation of food that is pure (which is directed to the spleen/pancreas) from that which is impure (which is directed to the large intestine and urinary bladder). The Small Intestine meridian plays the same role as the Heart meridian. It conveys food—whether physical food or psychological food—that is being processed, assuring assimilation on all levels. These transformations require a lot of heat, and that is why the small intestine belongs to the element Fire and why it represents the warmest spot in the body. In all other aspects it has the same physiological and psychological characteristics as the heart. The predominant solar time of the Small Intestine meridian is from 13:00 to 15:00 (1 p.m. to 3 p.m.).

The Heart Protector (Pericardium) Meridian

The pericardium is a double-walled sac containing the heart and the roots of the large vessels that bring blood to and from the heart. It is considered a virtual organ, one closely associated with the heart. Like the heart, it shares correspondences with the element Fire. The Heart Protector meridian, which is associated with the Chinese astrological sign of the Dog, helps the Heart meridian by controlling the central circulatory system, and in this way it helps regulate the nutrition of the body. Its body pathway ends at the tip of the middle finger on each hand. All relationships between the heart and the other organs must first transit through the Heart Protector (assisted by the Triple Heater) meridian. It tends to balance them. Its role is to transmit to the whole body the orders from the heart, the emperor, which is why Taoists call this meridian the "prime minister," the one in charge of connecting and balancing everything that takes place inside. It structures, constructs, ratifies, and legislates everything concerning our inner conceptualization of things, and it keeps an eye on inner markers and established beliefs. Finally, it is the one in charge of sexuality and the balancing of sexuality.

The Heart Protector is linked to the blood vessels for their structure, and to the myocardium and pericardium and the brain through its significant action on the mind and the quality of thought. It is in charge of keeping things moving and distributing things on both the physical plane (blood circulation) as well as the psychological plane (circulation of ideas, smooth-flowing thought, ability to recycle ideas). The emotions associated with it are joy, pleasure, and happiness. The predominant solar time of the Heart Protector is from 19:00 to 21:00 (7 p.m. to 9 p.m.).

The Triple Heater Meridian

This meridian is paired with the Heart Protector; its physiological correspondent is that of a viscus, and its Chinese astrological symbol is the Pig. Just as the Heart Protector is associated with the heart, the Triple Heater is associated with the small intestine. It corresponds to summer. Its body pathway begins at the tip of each ring finger. It assists the Small Intestine meridian and balances the energy provided by the Heart Protector, assisting it, but at a finer level—at the level of the capillaries and especially at the level of the lymph, while also having a specific action on the serous membranes, the layers of tissue that wrap around organs and help lubricate them so they don't get rubbed raw.

As its name indicates, the Triple Heater has a significant connection to heat. It controls the "atmosphere" in which the viscera work by regulating internal heat. It is the meridian that connects and balances the inner with everything coming from the outside. It structures, constructs, ratifies, and legislates everything about our conceptualization in relation to facts coming from the outside. It is the meridian that allows new markers of beliefs to become established in us.

On the physiological plane, each of the three planes of the Triple Heater are positioned at a different level in the body. The Upper Triple Heater corresponds to the part of the chest above the diaphragm; the Middle Triple Heater is associated with the part of the belly between the diaphragm and the navel; and the Lower Triple Heater corresponds to the belly below the navel. The predominant solar time of the Triple Heater is from 21:00 to 23:00 (9 p.m. to 11 p.m.).

Water

Urinary Bladder and Kidney Meridians

Water manages everything having to do with our deep energies. Like underground water, this is a powerful, deep energy that is in reserve and unchangeable. Ancestral energy is associated with the Water principle; it represents what is recorded in the deepest parts of ourself. These are our unconscious energies, our personal patterns on which we construct reality. Water corresponds to all our social, cultural, and family archetypes and all the unconscious memories that are recorded in us (in contrast with Earth, which represents our conscious memories and our store of experiences). Our deep, secret codes, such as what is recorded in our DNA, belong to the element of Water.

Of course, this bestows a phenomenal power on Water, which is why it is charged with our inner power, our resistance to effort, our capability for recuperation, and our deep will. Our energy reserves depend on Water as does our potential for longevity, which is linked to our ancestral energy. Our ability to decide, after having chosen (Metal) and gotten involved with things, as well as moving into action depends on Water. It is also present in our sense of listening and hearing, and in our ability to break down experiences so they can be integrated. By extension it relates to our potential for accepting things as they are, "going with the flow." On the psychological and mental level, severity, rigor, moving into action, and the sense of listening all depend on Water. Our deepest fears are also managed by this element.

Two meridians are associate with the Water principle, the Urinary Bladder meridian and the Kidney meridian.

The Urinary Bladder Meridian

The Urinary Bladder meridian is associated with winter, same as the Kidney meridian, with which it is complementary. Its pathway ends at the tip of each little toe on the feet, and it is associated with the Chinese astrological sign of the Monkey. This meridian is linked to the whole urinary apparatus as well as to the pituitary and the autonomic nervous system, which collaborate in stimulating secretion from the kidneys. The urinary bladder expels urine, the final product in the purification of organic fluids. This is the final phase in the transformation of energies since urine consists of impure fluids loaded with toxins and fluids that are in excess supply in the body. The bladder is coupled with the kidneys because it is the kidneys that direct the secretion of urine.

The bladder, along with the kidneys, supports the management and clearing of old memories, the old, deep patterns that all of us have been carrying around and that we are ready to change or let go of. This role is easily understood since these two meridians are closely connected with the autonomic nervous system, the physiological doorway to our nonconscious, which is precisely what carries our deepest memories.

The Urinary Bladder meridian corresponds to our bones, to the marrow of our bones, and to the ears. On the psychological level it is associated with severity, fecundity, rigor, and decisions, and to the sense of listening. Its predominant solar time is from 15:00 to 17:00 (3 p.m. to 5 p.m.).

The Kidney Meridian

The kidneys correspond to winter and are ruled by the Chinese astrological sign of the Rooster. The Kidney meridian begins on the ball of the foot. The kidneys control the composition and the secretion of organic fluids on which the life-force energy depends, and they manage our defense system against stress. They also regulate the body's acidity level and the quantity of toxins through their purification mechanisms. Finally, they direct the left and right adrenal glands, a role that accords them the management of our fears and reactive attitudes in confronting the world. Aggression, reactivity, the fight-or-flight instinct (adrenaline), or conversely tranquillity and our ability to quench what gets inflamed (corticosteroids) are managed by the kidneys based on their management of the adrenal glands.

The kidneys are in charge of storing water and any essential energy that hasn't been stored in any of the other organs for their own needs. In addition, they are the basis of the yin/yang balance of energy because life itself depends on the combination of Water and Fire in the kidneys. The left kidney is predominantly yang/Fire, whereas the right kidney is predominantly yin/Water. This laterality is very important and we will come back to it later in this book.

The kidneys are the very foundation of one's chi, or life force, and they participate notably in reproductive energy (fertility of the sperm and ova) through their yang/Fire character. Here we discover their relationship to the Heart Protector, which acts as their relay to the heart for everything connected to life and reproduction. The predominant solar time of the Kidney meridian is from 17:00 to 19:00 (5 p.m. to 7 p.m.).

Wood

Gall Bladder and Liver Meridians

The Wood principle corresponds to spring; it is therefore associated with the springtime of anything, that is, to its beginning. Our ability to get going with a project or an action, along with our imagination and creativity, depend on Wood. Wood represents birth and early child-hood. Our flexibility, our inner malleability and muscular tonicity, are managed by Wood. Like new growth sprouting from the earth after winter (the Water element), dreams depend on Wood because they are the expression of the nonconscious (Water). Wood allows us to travel, both inwardly and outwardly.

Everything connected with exteriorization (shouting, singing, but also theater and other forms of artistic expression) is managed by the energy of Wood. Our connection to aesthetics comes from this element. Shared love, respect for others, friendship, and faithfulness depend on it (in contrast to passionate love, which depends on Fire). The sense of ethics and respect for inner laws depends on Wood (whereas respect for outer laws is Metal). By extension and conversely, fear of betrayal and anger are also manifestations of this element when it is threatened or put off balance. Wood plays a significant role in the immunity that a person develops, on both the physiological and the psychological planes.

Two meridians are associated with the Wood principle, the Gall Bladder meridian and the Liver meridian.

The Gall Bladder Meridian

The gallbladder, like the liver, to which it is complementary, is associated with springtime. The Gall Bladder meridian ends in the fourth toe (the foot's "ring finger") and it is associated with the Chinese astrological sign of the Rat.

The gallbladder distributes nutritional elements and regularizes the energetic balance of the whole body. It directs the secretions of the glands in the digestive tract such as saliva, bile, and gastric, pancreatic, enteric, and duodenal secretions. It controls the harmonious and proper distribution of nutritional elements and works in close collaboration with the liver, which provides it with the basic elements for this work. This is why it is essential that the energy of the meridian pair Liver/Gall Bladder be balanced. Through its very nature the gall-bladder participates in the general attitude of the mind and that of the organs. If it is balanced, the mind and the organs will manage to address issues and will have the energy and the courage to resist challenges. If it is not sufficiently balanced, one's morale will be affected and a sense of defeat will enter and lay the groundwork for defeat to actually happen. In short, the gallbladder, along with its complementary organ, the liver, is in charge of everything concerning feelings and their effects. Since the gallbladder is yang, this association with feelings is connected with the exterior world and to the ability to live, experience, and express. There is also a connection with intuition and deep sincerity.

At a physiological level, this meridian, like the Liver meridian, corresponds to the eyes, the muscles, and the nails. On a psychological level the Gall Bladder meridian is associated with the sense of justice, courage, harmony, and purity. The predominant solar time of the Gall Bladder meridian is from 23:00 to 01:00 (11 p.m. to 1 a.m.).

The Liver Meridian

The Liver meridian begins on the top side of the tip of the big toe on each foot, the opposite side from the Spleen/Pancreas meridian; its Chinese astrological representation is the Ox. The liver supports the storage of nutritional elements, and through that it regulates the energy that supports general activity. It also determines our ability to resist illness by releasing the energy necessary for defense mechanisms in the case of the onset of illness. Finally, it plays a significant role in nourishment and in the decomposition and detoxification of the blood. This is where its role is active in relation to affecting feelings. In fact, the blood, which depends on the heart, transports emotions. If the blood is polluted, the quality of emotions will be bad and the feelings that they feed will also be of poor quality.

Because of its close connection with blood (in both production and composition), the liver plays a significant role in immune system processes. It drains away toxins, regulates coagulation, and regularizes the metabolism. Finally, it is the liver that determines the general quality of the energy. Like the gallbladder, it manages our connection to feelings, but in this case on a yin level, that is, in an inner way, by transforming, purifying, and filtering the emotions into feelings and their effects. The predominant solar time of the Liver meridian is from 01:00 to 03:00 (1 a.m. to 3 a.m.).

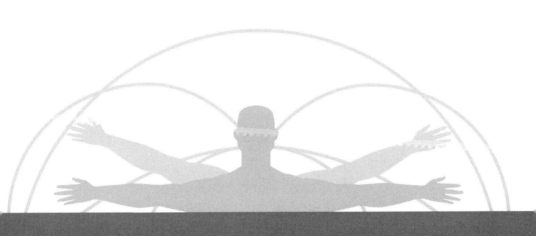

PART 2

A Symbolic Message System

How the Nonconscious Speaks through the Body

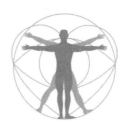

4

The Main Parts
of the Body

And How They Speak to Us

*The truths that we least want to hear are often those that
we most need to know.*

CHINESE PROVERB

How is the body put together, and what is the role of each of the organs
and organ systems that comprise it and support its existence and functioning in such a remarkably effective way? Now that we have established the basic theoretical framework of the Taoist understanding
of health and wellness, we are ready to discover what our aches and
pains are really trying to tell us. Understanding the subtle mechanisms
behind physical pain and discomfort allows us to see our symptoms in
a broader perspective—as signposts along life's path, and not as something foisted on us from some cruel external source. In this way we can
try to bring meaning to our pain rather than desperately seeking some
way to silence the signals that are trying to communicate something
much bigger and deeper to us.

As I made clear in the introduction to this book, I am not going to outline a systematic glossary in which you just look up "knee," for example, in order to be shown an exhaustive list of all the different interpretations of knee pain. There are already books out there that do just that. In my opinion this sidesteps the opportunity inherent in knowing the deeper significance of such pain, because the pain we experience in the knees or any other part of the body represents a message from the nonconscious, from one's own inner master. As in the case of dreams, the signs that pain sends us are always symbolic, and the strength of the pain varies in intensity according to the importance of the underlying problem. In the same way that no one can tell you the meaning of your dreams, no one can tell you what your troubles mean. I believe that all we can do is provide directions to ponder, frameworks for meaning, and not precise and clear-cut formulas that are valid for everyone. In the case of a woman who has pain in her left breast, I do not think you can say, for example (as I have read in certain books), "That means that you are not looking after yourself well enough" or "That means that you are too concerned about your children." These statements are partly true, but doubtless, also partly false. They allow those who deliver them to stay in a position of power, being those who "know," but they do not really provide the person with the possibility of evolving by finding out the deeper meaning on her own.

Each one of us carries within us a history that is our own and is unlike any other personal history. So then how can anyone generalize? In the case of the previous example, here is what I would suggest saying to this woman: "What do the breasts represent?" First, they are elements of femininity; next, they allow a child to be nourished, to be given food, a necessity of life. Therefore they represent two things: femininity, and the ability to look after others, taking care of them, and especially those whom we place or care for like a child. It is clear that during the period of breastfeeding and early childhood a woman forgets herself completely while mothering her offspring. She mothers and protects the child, who is completely dependent on her, in the same way that all those whom we mother or protect are dependent or become dependent on us. This latter kind of mothering sets up a power dynamic between the person doing the mothering and the person being mothered, under the pretext that the person cannot take care of himself or herself.

Again following this example, the woman's pain issue involves the left breast. Recall that left-handed laterality corresponds to yang, that is, to masculine symbolism. I would therefore ask this woman to consider which man is she is concerned about in an excessive way (husband, brother, boss, et al.), thinking of him as a child and forgetting herself in the process? Is she fleeing from the role of woman, preferring instead to be mother? Finally, I would ask her to reflect on the power dynamic inherent in her relationship with her man. Only the woman herself will be able to find the right answer within herself. Only she will be able to make this behavioral discovery so that she can choose to change her inner attitude. The presence of physical pain, illustrating that the situation does not suit her, will allow her to avoid going through a more serious illness and will focus her attention in such a way that it will facilitate the clearing of inner disharmony caused by her inappropriate mothering behavior.

In this way I will review the various organs and organ systems from the point of view of their psychological function, and not merely their mechanical structure. This gives us another perspective, one that is more open and intelligent as to the nature of our human experience.

Here I would like to once again touch on the subject of laterality in the body. Taoist philosophy has a very precise codification of energies. As we now know, right corresponds to yin and left to yang. There is a complete set of symbols associated with each of these energetic dynamics, as shown below. Anytime we find ourself in a lateralized manifestation in our body, we need to look at what is happening at that moment in our life (or in the recent past) in the affected area, proceeding in decreasing order of the degrees listed below, with the first degree carrying the most significant weight of meaning.

Yin Symbolism Right side of the body	Yang Symbolism Left side of the body
1st degree: mother, wife, daughter, sister	1st degree: father, husband, son, brother
2nd degree: women in general, femininity, the structure of things or of oneself, the right brain, feelings	2nd degree: man in general, masculinity, the personality of things or of oneself, the left brain, strength
Social degree: the family, the company (which represents the societal mother, the one that "nourishes and protects at her breast"), society, the church	Social degree: individualism, hierarchy (which represents the social father, he who educates, makes himself an example, or shows an example), authority figure, police

These correspondences of lateralities are also valid as a kind of basic self-diagnosis. In fact, we all have one side of the body that is dominant, from both a general perspective (flexibility, release in the hips or the foot, size of breast, etc.) and in the specifics (controlling eye, sensitivity of the ear, the side that you most often bump or hurt, etc.). This lateralization gives a general texture to our basic personal dynamic and tells us clearly whether it is yin (maternal representation) or yang (paternal representation) that predominates in us or with which we basically have something to "set right."

I must make clear a very important nuance that concerns the sense in which the messages need to be read and understood, and that is this: These messages are only meaningful when they exist, when they are expressed. They do not work systematically in reverse. They do not mean that such and such a problem, issue, or pain is going to necessarily exist because we are experiencing such and such a situation. If someone cries out, it means he is hurting. Conversely, it does not mean that if someone is hurting that he will necessarily cry out. Each person has her own threshold of expressing what she feels, but also her own preferred way of doing it. For example, among my clients I have two or three people who begin laughing uncontrollably when they are hurting, and believe me it is not because they like to suffer! Each time our leg hurts it means that we are experiencing tension in our relationships. But conversely, that does not mean that each time we are experiencing tension in our relationships that our leg is going to hurt. We can always choose, based on the reasons for this tension, another way or another place in which to express it—unless we know and simply choose to silence the tension.

The messages we receive from the body and the cries from the soul indicate that the truth lies within us; it is not outside us, nor is it defined by absolute criteria. That is why the meaning of the message functions in one direction only; it is not possible to say which behavior will inevitably lead to which illness or suffering in the body. The only truth that is transcendent, external, and imposed on us is the truth of the laws of life, the truth of the energetic balances that underlie life's manifestations. We have each chosen a portion of that truth in the Earlier Heaven; it can be summarized as: *Any thing or any attitude is bad when it is in excess.* This is why each one of the examples I cite in the following chapters is not intended to show or prove anything, but rather to illustrate and clarify. The rest is up to the individual reader. I do not ask you to believe me. I simply ask that you observe. You can then establish your own belief for yourself. I personally believe that in life success is not a matter of belief, but instead a matter of confidence. But when it comes to failure, that is always a problem of belief.

The Structure of the Human Body and the Role of Each Part

How is the body of each human being naturally put together? First, it is constructed around a frame, a solid, hard structure: the skeleton. This skeleton is rigid but jointed so that it supports all bodily movement. It is itself structured around a basic axis that is the spinal column, much the way a tree has a trunk from which all the branches extend outward.

Inside this load-bearing structure we have the various organs that find their places perfectly situated so that they function optimally. The whole is set in motion by a very extensive system of motors (muscles) and cables (tendons and ligaments). It is protected with an envelope (the skin) that completely encloses it. Staying with the bony structure, let's note how perfectly designed it is, such that the more important a part of the body is, the more vital and developed it is, the better it is protected by the skeleton.

The abdomen, which contains the viscera of digestion and elimination, is supported by the spinal column and rests on the pelvis but is not protected by a bony structure. It is supple, stretchable, and can move freely. The lungs and heart, which are even more vital, are also supported by the spinal column, but they are protected by the bony cage formed by the ribs. And although the ribs surround these essential organs they leave room for them to move around. Finally, we have the brain, which is entirely encased, protected in the strongbox of bone that is the cranium, the mobility of which, although existing in minute degrees (as all osteopaths know), is limited. As we can see, chance is absent when it comes to human construction—nothing is happenstance, and everything serves a purpose.

We are now ready to take each part of our body "machine" and study it in detail. This is how we are going to be able to find, for each part, the secret codes that will allow us to decipher the underlying messages our body sends us.

The Skeleton and the Spinal Column

The spinal column is made up of vertebrae, each one of which plays a very precise role. They number five for the sacral vertebrae, five for the lumbar vertebrae, twelve for the thoracic vertebrae, and seven for the cervical vertebrae. Here we can begin to appreciate the logic in the construction of the human body. The number 5 carries much symbolism, both for the human being and for matter in general (the Five Principles, five senses, five fingers, etc.). There are five sacral and lumbar vertebrae, which make up the two bases of our spinal column (one fixed, the "source," and the other mobile, the "base"). The number 7 symbolizes spirituality, the divine, what is highly developed (seven chakras, seven

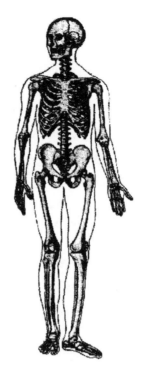

Fig. 4.1. The skeleton

colors of the rainbow, seven branches of the Jewish candelabra, etc.). The cervical vertebrae, which carry what is most developed in us, namely, the head, number seven. Finally, the thoracic vertebrae, which support the upper body, are twelve in number, which is the sum of the two (5 + 7 = 12), a number reflected in the twelve signs of the zodiac, the twelve months of the year, the twelve hours of the day, the twelve homeopathic salts, the twelve Apostles, and so forth. I find it very hard to believe that these numbers are based only on chance.

Each vertebra has a specific role and serves as a distribution center for vibratory data coming from the brain. Both the conscious and the nonconscious communicate with the body through the mechanical and chemical support of the central computer that is the brain. It transmits its instructions to the smallest of our cells, notably through the cerebrospinal nervous system and the autonomic nervous system

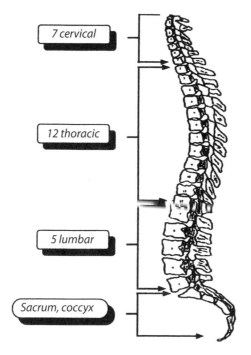

7 cervical

12 thoracic

5 lumbar

Sacrum, coccyx

Fig. 4.2. The spinal column

(the sympathetic and parasympathetic systems). According to the type of tension and its intensity, a process of clearing any excess energy is produced in the area of the vertebra.

For example, a muscular contraction around a vertebra will first engender the sensation of pain of varying intensity. If the imbalance persists or if the pain is silenced with medication or other palliative techniques, the problem very often worsens and changes into arthrosis (i.e., osteoarthritis), a herniated disc, or some other form of organic dysfunction. Notably, this phenomenon happens—or rather is discovered—very often upon awakening in the morning, that is, right after nighttime. Nighttime is the favorite period for there to be activity and expression from our nonconscious. The inner master needs the silence of the night to speak because the tumult and agitation of the day make it impossible to be heard. The noise of the carriage on the road and the fact that the master is seated inside means that the coachman and the master can only converse after they have stopped, at pauses chosen or caused by some event along the way.

It is only in the most "urgent" or "intense" cases that we need to resort to a slipped disc, with which we're going to make exactly the right move to "immobilize" our back. A detailed explanation of the main disc slippages is relatively easy to work out using the following table, which shows us a little bit about the connections between each of the vertebrae and the organs.

Cervical vertebrae	Distribution center for	Standard symptoms
1st cervical	Head, face, sympathetic system	Headache, insomnia, depression, dizziness
2nd cervical	Eyes, hearing, sinus, tongue	Dizziness, seeing or hearing problems, allergies
3rd cervical	Face, ears, teeth	Acne, red patches, eczema, toothache
4th cervical	Nose, lips, mouth	Allergies (hay fever, cold sores, etc.)
5th cervical	Neck and throat	Infection and pain in throat
6th cervical	Muscles of the neck, shoulders, upper arms	Torticollis (stiff neck), shoulder pain
7th cervical	Shoulders, elbows, little fingers, and ring fingers	Pain, itching, and swelling in these areas

Thoracic vertebrae	Distribution center for	Standard symptoms
1st thoracic	Forearms, hands, wrists, thumbs, index and middle fingers, carriage of the head	Pain, itching, and swelling in these areas
2nd thoracic	Cardiac system, cardiac plexus	Cardiac symptoms or pain
3rd thoracic	Pulmonary system, breasts	Pulmonary disease, pain in breasts

Thoracic vertebrae	Distribution center for	Standard symptoms
4th thoracic	Gallbladder	Gallbladder attacks, morale, certain gallbladder-related migraines, and cutaneous infections
5th thoracic	Hepatic system, solar plexus	Issues with the liver or immune system, emotional fragility
6th thoracic	Digestive system, stomach, solar plexus	Digestive issues, gastric acidity, air swallowing
7th thoracic	Spleen/pancreas	Diabetes
8th thoracic	Diaphragm	Hiccups, pain in solar plexus
9th thoracic	Adrenals	Aggression, reactivity, allergic reactions
10th thoracic	Kidneys	Poor elimination, food poisoning, intoxication, tire easily
11th thoracic	Kidneys	Poor elimination, food poisoning, intoxication, tire easily
12th thoracic	Small intestine, lymphatic system	Poor assimilation, joint pain, gas

Lumbar vertebrae	Distribution center for	Standard symptoms
1st lumbar	Large intestine	Constipation, colitis, diarrhea
2nd lumbar	Abdomen, thighs	Cramps, abdominal pain
3rd lumbar	Sex organs, knees	Painful menstrual periods, impotency, cystitis, knee pain
4th lumbar	Sciatic nerve, lumbar muscles	Sciatica, lumbar pain, urination problems
5th lumbar	Sciatic nerve, lower legs	Cramps, lower legs heavy, painful, sciatica
Sacrum and coccyx	Pelvis, buttocks, spine	Spinal problems, sacroiliac problems, hemorrhoids

Skeletal and Spinal Issues

The skeleton and the bones represent our structure, our inner architecture. Whenever we suffer in the bones it means that we are suffering in our inner structures, in our life beliefs. Most of these structures are unconscious. They are our deepest archetypes, and we continually depend on them without our conscious awareness in our day-to-day life and in our relationship to life. The broad area of the beliefs of peoples (history, culture, customs, religions) form part of these archetypes, including those beliefs that are more personal such as racism, ethics, a sense of honor or justice, perversions, or gut fears. Our bones are what are deepest in our body, around which everything else is built, on which our body rests and finds support. The bones are also what are hardest, most rigid, and solid in us. In the pith of the bones the bone marrow, the "inner philosopher's stone," where the most secret human alchemy takes place, is sheltered. The bones and the bone marrow represent what is deepest in us: they form the basis of our nonconscious psychology. In short, our relationship to life is built on and around our bones.

When we are deeply upset, affected, or touched to the quick in our deep, fundamental beliefs as they relate to life or as they relate to what we believe life is or should be, our bone structure will express that to us with pain and discomfort. This is why **osteoporosis** develops among certain (but not all) women after menopause—because frequently at this stage of life a woman experiences menopause as a loss of feminine identity. The deep, archetypal image of that woman is of one who procreates. In fact, for many women "mother" has for a long time been her only social role. Traditionally, sterile or menopausal women have been considered useless both to the community and to the family, to the point where they were frequently repudiated by their husbands.

Generalized attacks on the bony structure are rare and most often are confined to a precise location in the body (leg, arm, head, wrist, etc.). In each case the meaning of the message behind the pain is directly related to the location, while taking into account the fact that the problem expressed in that spot is deep, structural, and linked to a fundamental belief that rightly or wrongly has been disturbed by what the person is going through.

Scoliosis is a striking example of a structural issue. It is a deformation of the spine that can be very serious and has specific characteristics. It affects children usually during the preteen years and usually stops after puberty. Let us see now how it's possible to understand simply and clearly the mechanism and symbolism of scoliosis. A child's developmental phase is the time in which he heads toward adulthood (at least in physical form), a time when he leaves the world of childhood. The phenomenon of scoliosis occurs during this time when the spine is growing between two defined axes, the pelvis and the shoulders. The two poles remain at an equal distance apart, while the top one stays at the same distance from the ground. This causes a sideways curve in the spine.

What does this represent for the child, and what is the meaning of this growth pattern that cannot be discerned from the outside? The shoulders, which are the yang axis of the body, the axis of action (see the section on the shoulders and arms later in this chapter), are the representation of the father, while the hips, which are the yin axis of the body, the axis of relationship (see the section on the hips in this chapter), are the representation of the mother. These are the two unconscious spatial orientation points that the child has about his place and that of his parents, whether his actual parents or his symbolic parents (teachers, guardians, et al.). If the adult world is not satisfactory to the child, his desire to displace his own orientation points in order to join theirs will disappear, and the child will reject this unattractive world. He will then unconsciously choose to remain in the world of childhood, which suits him better. He thus freezes the external orientation points of his growth, those that he sees and can measure. The lines of the shoulders and pelvis will then stay at the same height, at the same distance apart. However, the spine continues to grow and is thus obliged to develop between these two fixed points, resulting in curvature. Sometimes a serious increase of curvature develops. When this happens we say that the scoliosis has "flared up."

The second characteristic of scoliosis is that it always stops at the end of puberty. Puberty represents the period when the child is calibrating his emotional life in relation to the external world, when he is verifying his ability to find his place and be loved and recognized externally. Once he has found this place, he no longer needs to freeze his orientation points and can allow them to move once again.

I am thinking very much here about Carine. This young girl, aged fourteen, had a problem with a flare-up of scoliosis, at which point the specialists urgently advised her parents that she wear a rigid corset that enclosed the whole of her torso 24/7, and to do that for a minimum of several months. Her father, who was seeing me for problems with his own sciatica, spoke to me about Carine. After advising him to seek several medical opinions before doing anything, I explained to him what was likely behind his daughter's scoliosis. I also proposed helping the girl understand what was happening and how she could change this "bad programming," which was making her unhappy. As well, I advised her to seek the help of a homeopathic doctor as well as a professional friend who practices a technique called ortho-bionomy, a gentle, noninvasive system of healing that reminds the body of its natural ability to restore balance. In the following months, Carine stopped cold the progress of her scoliosis (which had cost her one or two degrees) and began growing again (three to four centimeters), which she had not done for a year.

What was happening in Carine's life to bring on the scoliosis? In the year preceding her visit to my office she had lost all her stable markers or guidelines as a result of decisions made by adults. The family had moved, so she had to change schools, and the totally absorbing professional activities of her father, who seemed to her to be absent too often, caused her to lose faith in the adult world. Carine still had one ray of sunshine in her heart—the deep friendship of a girlfriend at school who was very dear to her. However, she once again was betrayed by adults because the parents of this girl decided to move, and the girl's mother refused to allow the two girls to see each other from time to time or even engage in correspondence. From that day on, Carine stopped growing and decided to hang on to her childhood markers. I knew that Carine had won the battle when after our third session she recounted how the night preceding our session she had a nightmare in which a "murderer killed a child."

The Lower Limbs

Let's now take a look at how our body is constructed, clothed, and jointed. Starting at the bottom, we have the lower limbs, the trunk, the upper limbs, and the head. Each one of these body parts plays a very precise role that is directly related to its function. We will be concentrating on the exact functions of each part, whether a limb or an organ.

The lower limbs are composed of two parts, the upper leg (thigh and femur), and the lower leg (calf, tibia, and fibula), and the three important axes that are their main joints. The lower limbs end in a masterful structure: the foot.

The joints that connect and articulate the foot, the lower leg, the upper leg, and the torso are the hips, the knees, and the ankles. What is the primary physiological role of the legs? They allow us to move about, to go forward or backward, from one place to another, and, of course,

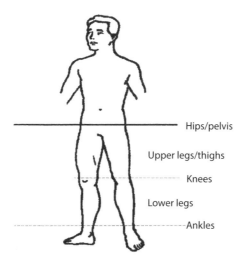

Hips/pelvis

Upper legs/thighs

Knees

Lower legs

Ankles

Fig. 4.3. The lower limbs

toward or away from other people and things. Therefore, they are our mobility agents that put us in relationship with the world and with others. The societal symbolism of the legs is very strong. It's the legs that make it possible to have gatherings, meetings, contacts, and movement forward. Everything belonging to the legs is connected to movement in space, notably in the space of relationships. Our legs then are our agents of relationship, whether it is in their role in psychological representation or in their potential as physical agents.

Lower Limb Issues

In a general sense, when we have tension or pain in the legs it means that we have tension in our relationship with the world or with someone; we are having difficulty moving forward or backward in the relational space of the moment. The more precisely we can pinpoint the location within the leg, the more we will be able to refine the type of tension we are experiencing and the more likely we will understand it. In this discussion we will be going into detail about the specific meaning of each part of the leg. Bear in mind that we have to always position any kind of leg issue within the basic framework, which is that of relationship with the world and with others. Let's first look at the joints of the leg: the hips, knees, and ankles; then we'll go on to the thigh, the calf, and the foot.

▸ THE HIPS

The hips are the primary "mother" joint of the lower limbs. It is from the hips that all potential movement of the lower limbs begins. The hips also represent the basic axis of our world of relationships. They are the doorway of the relational nonconscious (see figure 4.4 on page 114), that is, the point through which the elements of our nonconscious emerge and move toward the conscious. Our deepest patterns, our beliefs about relating to others and to the world and our subsequent experiences of the world are somatically represented in the body's structure by the hips. Any disturbance, whether conscious or not, of these areas in life will have repercussions in one or both of the hips. Along with the pelvis and the lumbar area, the hips are the seat of our deep strength as well as a source of mobility that symbolizes inner and outer flexibility. It is based on our hips that our being is in relationship with the world.

Hip Issues

Problems with the hips—pain, tension, blockages, arthrosis, etc.—show us that we are moving through a situation where the basis of our deeply held beliefs is being brought into question. That this joint, which is the primary, fundamental support for the leg, lets go means that our deep inner supports, our most deeply rooted beliefs connecting us to life, are letting go as well. We are experiencing betrayal or abandonment, whether our own or someone else's.

If it's a matter of the left hip, we have the case of an experience of treason or abandonment with yang (paternal) symbolism. I'm thinking here of Sylvie, who came to see me about a problem of arthrosis in her left hip just before having it operated on. After letting her speak about her mechanical suffering in the hip, I led her to the heart of the problem. I encouraged her to talk a little more about her life, asking her, "Which man betrayed you or let you down in these last few months?" Much surprised by my question, she confided that her husband had abandoned her three years earlier, but she didn't see any connection between this event and her hip problem. I explained that the unconscious process had taken all that time to release this loss. She then realized that indeed she had experienced the disappearance of her husband as an abandonment and something that was unfair. After two sessions of harmonization massage and work on this memory, her hip released to the point that by the following week she was able to experience two complete days without feeling the slightest pain. Her fears and her professional obligations compelled her nonetheless to undergo the operation, and of course I made it clear to her that the choice was hers. The operation was a complete success and completely silenced her pain.

A year and a half later Sylvie came back to see me for the same problem, this time with her right hip. It was clear that she had released none of the previous internal tension she had recounted in her earlier sessions with me. The wound in her soul had not healed at all; it merely migrated to another point in her body where it could be expressed. I pushed her further to speak about her experience, and finally she confessed that after the disappearance of her husband she suspected that he had cheated on her, so as his wife she naturally felt betrayed. It was not surprising that her nonconscious needed to announce her inner wound via her hip. This time, however, it was the right hip, her yin side; her femininity had surely suffered from this betrayal, and because she had had the left hip fixed through surgical means it could no longer "speak," so the job had been taken up by the right hip.

When the right hip is involved we have a case of an experience of betrayal or abandonment of yin (maternal) symbolism. This reminds me of my own father. He worked in a government office where the way people behaved became increasingly intolerable to him because they had betrayed the concept he had of what public service should be. How can one escape such a situation? One day he had a fall in which he hurt his right hip very badly. Little by little, his pain increased to the point where it became physically difficult for him to do his work. Being a country person and having a strong sense of duty and respect for commitments, he was even more frustrated when it was suggested that he take sick leave. "I can't accept that because it would mean that others will have to do my work in my place," he said at the time. That would have been an additional betrayal, but this time his own. To avoid it he took early retirement, even though in doing so he took a financial hit because he was not far from full retirement. However, he was not able to understand the complete unconscious significance of what was happening.

After he retired from his government job he helped someone he knew create a trout-farming operation. The beginning seemed promising, but the experience of betrayal happened again. The person he was working with began to jab him daily with "jokes" that belittled his contribution to the work. One day the jokes became too much for him to bear. The pain in his right hip, which had taken the form of a hip-based arthrosis, flared up to such an extent that he had to undergo an operation.

This was twenty-five years ago. Perhaps if I had known at the time what I know now, we could have evoked his need to experience the betrayal or symbolic abandonment. He had already encountered abandonment and betrayal when he was younger. Returning home after being imprisoned during the war he realized that his father had abandoned the beautiful farm where he had lived before the war. He had deliberately exhorted his father not to do that. Realizing that his father had sold it anyway so he could buy another one somewhere else, he decided then to leave the family farm and take a job in a factory. I say "perhaps" because we are not always ready to hear certain things, and no one can experience or change another person's Life Path.

▶ THE KNEES

The knees are the second joints of the legs that are used to bend and to kneel. This is the gesture of humility, inner suppleness, and deep strength—the opposite of external force, which makes for rigidity. It is the manifest sign of allegiance, acceptance, or even surrender and submission; thus it represents the doorway of acceptance (see figure 4.4 on page 114). The knees are continuations of the hips, and they prolong their mobility, but in the opposite direction inasmuch as the hips can only bend forward while the knees can only bend backward. Therefore they stand for the ability to let go, cede, or even back up. They are also the joints that swing between the conscious and the nonconscious. They represent the acceptance of a deep feeling or an idea that emerges from the nonconscious toward the conscious if we are in the process of densification; conversely, they also represent a movement toward the nonconscious from the conscious if we are in the process of liberation (as shown in figure 4.4). The knees are the major joints of relating to others and represent our ability to accept what that relationship implies in the way of opening or even compromising (I do not mean debasing yourself, though).*

Knee Issues

It's fairly easy to see that when we have a knee problem it means that we are having difficulty bending to or accepting a particular experience. Because we are dealing with the legs, the tension is along the lines of relationship with the external or internal world, with others or with oneself. Pain or mechanical problems with the knees mean that an emotion, a deep feeling, an idea, or a memory connected to our relationship with the world is not accepted or is even rejected. There is something that has been experienced in the conscious that has upset, turned around, or disturbed our inner beliefs, and we are rejecting it. Or the problem can involve an emotion, a deep feeling, or a memory that emerges from the nonconscious that we have difficulty accepting and integrating into our day-to-day life, into our conscious, because what is emerging disturbs or upset habits or beliefs that are known and established.

If it's the right knee, the tension is related to yin (maternal) symbolism. Here we might recall the example I referred to earlier of the man who hurt his right knee during a soccer match after he was served with divorce papers by his wife, something he had previously refused to agree to. I am thinking also of a personal example that is similarly meaningful.

A few years ago I was training very hard in aikido with my teacher at that time. With our blood, sweat, and tears, a few friends and I had built a magnificent dojo in Paris. In the process we had jeopardized our family and social obligations because this building project had taken precedence over everything else and made us unavailable for many other things. Shortly after the end of the building project, of which we were

---

*Translator's note: Notably, the French word for knee, *genou,* can be written phonetically as *je-nous,* meaning "I-us."

particularly proud, the relationships within the structure of the aikido association began to fall apart. But in my depths I could not accept the messages that kept coming to me, showing me that my time with the aikido association was over. It was too difficult for me to accept this idea after all that I had invested in it, despite the experience of betrayal that was connected to the ending.

It was my right knee that gave way and obliged me to stop the whole thing—the courses I was giving as well as the ones I was taking. I sustained a double sprain in an almost casual fashion during an aikido warm-up after my knee had already been hurting for several weeks. At the time I was unable to hear the message that my relationship with the association and its family dynamic was coming to an end. This new tension, added to the tension produced in my own family environment during the construction of the dojo, led to the sprain, while at the same time I injured my right hip (the experience of betrayal). This is how I was obliged to leave the association, a maternal representation. After thinking hard about it, I finally understood the message. Despite the medical seriousness of my injuries, I was able to quickly take up my aikido practice elsewhere; not so surprisingly, my right knee returned to perfect shape, allowing me to do aikido again, although the amount of time I spend on it now is not as extensive.

If it's a question of the left knee, the tension is related to yang (paternal) symbolism. Here I will take a young woman, Françoise, as an example. She came to see me complaining that she was feeling generally out of sorts. During our conversation it emerged that her left knee was hurting. To my question as to whether she was experiencing tension in a relationship with a man, and after looking at me as if I were a sorcerer, she admitted that she was going through a difficult period with her boyfriend in which she was no longer willing to accept his behavior. I then explained to her how the tension in her knee was related to the tension in her relationship with her boyfriend. After a few seconds of reflecting on that, she exclaimed, "My goodness! That's true because a few years ago I was living with another man with whom I had the same problem, and I also had sharp pain in my left knee that stopped shortly after we split up." I suggested to her that she should think about why she was reliving the same experience and why her body was sounding the alarm bell. This is how we were able to quickly resolve her "un-ease."

▸ THE ANKLES

The ankles are the third and last major joints in the legs and provide mobility between the feet and the legs. These major joints enable a range of motion to the mobility of the leg, notably when the foot is stationary, placed on the ground, or in motion. It is thanks to the ankles that we can "push" on our grounding support, the feet, to move forward better and faster.

While the hip represents the basic hinge of the unconscious structures and orientation points in relationships, the ankles (at the other end of the leg) signify the final, exteriorized hinge, the conscious orientation point. This joint supports our relationship to the world. It is the hinge in our beliefs in relation to others and to ourself. It symbolizes the ability to make decisions and changes in life and to involve ourself in things. The ankle is the doorway of involvement, as shown in figure 4.4 on page 114, in the sense of decision-making. Ground symbolizes reality; therefore the stability and mobility of our ground support (as well as its suppleness and its gentleness) depends on the ankles. This means the ankles are a faithful projection of rigidity or flexibility in our positions and in our life standards.

Ankle Issues

Pain or trauma in the ankles speaks about relationship difficulties in the sense that we lack stability or flexibility in those relationships. Ankle issues mean that the way in which we have positioned ourself in relation to life and to others doesn't work anymore, doesn't satisfy us anymore. Ankle issues force us to stop because we can no longer go on in the same way with others. The position that we are holding is not right for us; it is not realistic or is too rigid, and therefore we need to change our point of support, which consists of a belief we are holding. Pain in the ankles can also mean that we are having difficulty deciding something or making an important decision in life, no doubt because doing so risks bringing into question a current position or belief.

If the pain is in the right ankle it is related to the yin (maternal) dynamic. I am thinking here of a client named Peter. He came to see me about pain in his right ankle and in the right Achilles tendon. Being a keen jogger, this bothered him a lot as it was preventing him from enjoying his favorite way of unwinding and relaxing. His wife was a nervous, anxious person, and she had unintentionally created tension in the family dynamic, especially with their two daughters. Peter was having more and more difficulty accepting this situation and no longer knew which way to turn (an ankle metaphor), what position he should take with his wife so that she could find a way to calm down. Peter was also experiencing tension at work. His business was restructuring and he didn't know what his attitude was in relation to the changes that were being implemented. Two important axes of the yin dynamic, as represented by Peter's relationship with his wife and with his business, were being called into question.

If it's the left ankle, the tension is related to the yang (paternal or fraternal) dynamic. That's what happened in the case of Jacques and Françoise, two clients, both of whom had twisted their left ankles. In Jacques's case his boss, an old man and father figure, wasn't able to pass the baton to the next generation of leadership, and Jacques didn't know how to address this issue with him. In the case of Françoise, it turned out her son was taking drugs, something she had a lot of trouble admitting to herself, and she didn't know what attitude she should she should have toward him and toward the external world.

▶ **THE FOOT**

The foot is our point of support on the ground on which the whole body rests as well as the support point for all locomotion. It allows us to push forward and therefore to advance, but also to plant our support and "stand our ground." The foot represents the extremity of how our relationship with the external world manifests. It symbolizes our attitudes, our affirmed and recognized positions, and the official role we play. Do we stick our foot in the door to block it from closing? Do we stick our foot in our mouth from time to time?

The foot also represents one's standards and ideals. It is the symbolic key to what supports our relationships, which explains the significance of the rite of washing the feet in so many traditions. It is that which purifies our relationship to the world, and even to the divine. Finally, the foot is the symbol of freedom since it allows movement. It is not by chance that the feet of young Chinese girls were bound. Disguised as an erotic or aesthetic practice, it in fact signified that in traditional Chinese society a woman's mobility was limited and that women were essentially imprisoned in their relationship to men and society. But this isn't just a phenomenon of the East, as basically the same thing is found in the West, in the practice of women wearing very high heels to conform to certain ideas about femininity and women's place in the world. At least the feminist movement made it possible for more and more women to throw away their high heels and adopt more sensible footwear.

Foot Issues

Foot problems express the tension that we feel connected to our position as we face the world. It may concern our habitual attitudes, the unrealistic positions that we have taken on, or a lack of stability or security. The expression "He doesn't have his feet firmly planted on the ground" illustrates this kind of situation. When someone holds back or is uncomfortable in his position we say that "he hasn't yet found his footing" in the situation. Or if someone has chosen an unfortunate attitude in relation to another person we say that he has "gotten off on the wrong foot" with that person.

When pain manifests in the right foot it is related to yin (mother), and when it occurs in the left foot it is related to yang (father). Here

Judith comes to mind. This child of nine was brought in to see me by her mother because she was suffering from reflex neurovascular dystrophy of the ankle and left foot. The medical profession had predicted that the girl would end up in a wheelchair. This condition, especially deep and known to be of somatic origin, is sometimes so painful that it can lead people to suicide. What was happening in little Judith's life? She had just lost her father to a violent death. During the last part of his life Judith's father drank heavily. A couple of weeks before his death Judith began to feel pain in her left ankle. The girl no longer knew what she could depend on and lacked a father, the symbol of the pillar of strength. This manifested as the demineralizing of her ankle—her ankle was literally crumbling. We worked together to de-dramatize and reconstruct her emotional memory and to rebalance her energies. In addition, given the urgency and seriousness of the girl's condition, I immediately referred her to a homeopathic practitioner who conducted a deep remineralization treatment, as well as to a friend who helped her with sessions of ortho-bionomy. At the end of two weeks Judith was able to set aside her crutches and return to school—to the great surprise of the school doctor who accused the child of faking it since how else could she be walking again? It took me two more sessions to counteract a recurrence, which no doubt was the result of the girl having to encounter the negative attitude of yet another male authority figure.

▶ TOES

Toes are the fingers of the feet. They represent the fine endings, the details, the finishing touches of these important points of grounding and support. They therefore correspond to the end points of our positions, the details of our beliefs, or the punctuation of our relational attitudes. Each toe represents a particular detail, a specific mode or phase that we decipher thanks to the energetic meridian that ends or begins in the given toe. Because of their role as symbols of the peripheral, finishing elements in relationships, it is easy for a person to use the toes as a means of feedback. Thanks to the energetic points at the tip of each toe, the individual can stimulate or clear unconsciously but effectively the possible tensions that are found there. Both the toes and the fingers are places where we seem to experience random and seemingly meaningless little slipups in the form of bumps, burns, bruises, or cuts. However, it is never in fact random that we hurt such and such a toe or finger. In every case there is an underlying message about tension in a relationship. This is because the energy point that is at the tip of each one of the toes (and fingers) is a "source point" or "springtime point." It is the point of a possible rebirth of energy, thanks to which a new dynamic can appear, and by which the old one can "recharge" and change polarity.

Issues with the Toes

The following is a concise summary of the overall meaning of each of the toes and what is expressed if any one of them is in pain. Keep in mind that there is a distinct energetic meridian that ends at each toe, which represents a specific dynamic. Beyond that, if pain manifests in a toe of the right foot, it relates to yin (maternal) symbolism; if in a toe of the left foot, yang (paternal) symbolism is trying to express itself.

The big toe (the "thumb" of the foot): This is the only toe where two energetic meridians begin: the Spleen/Pancreas and the Liver meridians. This is the base toe of our relational support and of who and what we are. It is for this reason that during menopause women frequently develop **bunions,** a deformation in the big toe (known as *hallux valgus*); this is related to the loss of fertility, which often brings a sense of losing one's feminine value. Trauma or tension in this toe means that we are feeling an equivalent tension in our relationship to the world, whether on the material plane (inner side of the foot) or the affective plane (outer side of the foot).

The second toe (the "index finger" of the foot): This toe includes the Stomach meridian, which manages our connection to matter and our digestion of matter. Blisters, calluses, aches, or trauma to this "finger of the foot" is speaking to us about our difficulty managing certain material or professional situations.

The third toe (the "middle finger" of the foot): Though there is no organic meridian in this toe, it is indirectly related to the Triple Heater. It is therefore the central toe, the one related to the balance and coherence of our relational attitudes. Troubles with or aches in this toe mean that we are having trouble balancing our relationships, specifically as they relate to the future. Fear of moving forward and in the right way is expressed by this toe.

The fourth toe (the "ring finger" of the foot): This is the toe where the Gall Bladder meridian terminates. It represents the details of our relationship with the world, in the sense of just and unjust, and the search for perfection. When we have tension, cramps, or aches in this toe, it means that we are experiencing a difficult relational situation in terms of just or unjust. It's a question of a relationship that does not satisfy us with respect to the conditions and the quality of those conditions.

The little toe (the "little finger" of the foot): This is where the Urinary Bladder meridian ends. This is the meridian responsible for clearing the body of fluids, i.e., old memories. When we bang this toe—which is extremely painful as most of us who have done this know—we are trying to get rid of old memories, old habits, or old patterns of relating to the world and to others, patterns that no longer bring us any satisfaction. By means of trauma or pain in this area we are stimulating our energy to facilitate the clearing away of old modes of thinking and behaving so that they can be replaced with new and more effective modes.

▶ THE THIGHS AND FEMUR

The thighs are located between the hips and the knees. Recall that the hips and pelvis are representations of the relational unconscious;

specifically, they represent the gateway to the nonconscious, the gateway of integration, the point of emergence or resurgence of our nonconscious in relation to the world and to beings (including ourself). The knee, as I have said, is the doorway or demarcation line of acceptance, allegiance, or even surrender and submission. The thighs, built around the femur bone, represent what is between the two and what connects them. It may involve the transit phase of memories, fears, or desires moving from the nonconscious to the conscious, indicating a process of densification of energy (see figure 4.4) at the moment that precedes conscious acceptance. However, it can also work in reverse, as a process transiting from the conscious to the nonconscious. In that case it is a process of liberation, the moment that follows conscious acceptance and that precedes nonconscious acceptance.

Issues with the Thighs and the Femur

Deep, unconscious memories or wounds that one refuses to accept will manifest as tension (sore points, cramps, localized sciatic pain, etc.) in the thigh. These kinds of memories may manifest as a fracture of the femur when the memory is too strong or upsets the structure (the bone) of one's personal beliefs or life choices. On the other hand, pain here can involve tribulations and experiences that the person has accepted consciously, in his thinking, but that he hasn't been able to accept or is not yet ready to accept in the deepest part of himself. This can be someone who has had to give up something (societal promotion, work, home, country), which he understands and accepts in his mind, yet in the deepest part of himself he does not accept it. Despite all the logical reasons that have allowed him to understand things, he nevertheless can't integrate on an unconscious level. If the pain or the trauma is located in the femur, it means that the tension is connected to the deep structure, to the unconscious beliefs and values of the person. If it is located in the thigh, in the muscles themselves, we are dealing with a manifestation that is less serious since it is less anchored in the structure.

If the tension, pain, or fracture is located in the right thigh, it is yin-related and connected to maternal symbolism. Here I am thinking of a friend who for certain economic reasons had to sell his house. He knew it was necessary and even unavoidable. This need was clear in his head, and he had mentally accepted all the reasons for doing so when we spoke about it in casual conversation. The only problem was that for several years he had been providing living space for his mother in part of the house, and it was impossible for him to even imagine telling her that he was the one who was going to have to sell the house and that she was going to have to leave. The resulting tension was expressing itself in repeated and sometimes violent bouts of pain that moved around his right buttock, his right thigh, and his right knee. This reflected his psychological state and his degree of inner acceptance.

If on the other hand the tension, pain, or fracture is in the left thigh, it is yang-related, connected to paternal symbolism. This was the case with Pascal. At the age of only sixteen months he fractured his left femur. The circumstances were not sufficiently clear in his memory, so it is difficult to determine what was behind this fracture, which is very rare at such a young age. Then he lost his father to a traffic accident several years later. After that Pascal refused to "see" things, and so he manifested a serious problem in his left eye—a problem that disappeared almost overnight when the doctors decided to perform exploratory surgery because the examinations showed no pathology or lesions. It is clear that Pascal's relationship with paternal symbolism—meaning hierarchy, authority, and how he saw himself as a man—was unconsciously affected by his father's sudden death. Later in life Pascal experienced a difficult situation of affective failure in his life as a man, and once again he fractured his left femur in a traffic accident. The accident led his family to realize the depth of his long-denied distress. The painful memory was simply too strong to be acknowledged, and so it expressed itself in him fracturing his femur. Living from day to day, Pascal let his life drift along, seemingly giving in to a suicidal inner programming that was well underway. Having come to the end of the road, he finally decided to go into therapy to stop this dysfunctional dynamic and to pull himself together. Everything shifted when he did. He met the woman who was to become his wife, and he rebuilt his image of himself as a man. This occurred when he was thirty-four years old—exactly the same age his father was when he disappeared.

▶ THE CALF, THE TIBIA, AND THE FIBULA

These three areas of the body are located between the knee and the ankle. The knee, as we know, is the doorway of acceptance, while the ankle is the doorway of decision, that is, the point of transition in the world of status and property. When we have a new idea that comes from the depths of our nonconscious, and when we have accepted it (the knee), we must integrate it into our conscious concepts of relating to the world, into our life standards and our ideals of life. If this integration is difficult, there will be tension in the calves in the form of cramps or pain, or a fracture of the tibia and/or fibula.

This is the part of the body that precedes or follows the foot according to whichever way the energy is circulating, whether densifying or liberating. If moving through memories, fears, desires, or experiences from the nonconscious to the conscious (from the knee to the foot), it is a process of densification. This occurs at the moment following conscious acceptance of the painful memories, preceding their integration. Conversely, it can be movement from the conscious to the nonconscious (from the foot toward the knee). This is a process of liberation that precedes nonconscious acceptance and follows conscious acceptance of these memories, fears, or desires in the real world.

Issues in the Calves, Tibia, and Fibula

These three areas of the body speak to us about our difficulty accepting changes in our personal standards that are imposed by what we are going through in life. Difficulties in changing our opinion or our position on a habitual point of view in our relationship to the world can manifest through pain in this part of the leg. Fracture can occur when the tension is strong enough and when our position is so firmly entrenched that it cannot permit change imposed from the outside. In such a case it is the tibia or the fibula, or even both, that will let go and break. But even simple stiffness in the calf is telling us that we are having trouble budging off a fixed reference point or support in life, allowing the ankle and foot to engage in their role of mobility. This is also when **sciatica** manifests, as the lower leg tries to express that we are being rigid about something.

If the tension manifests in the left calf it is yang-related, connected to paternal dynamics. Take the example of Clotilde, who was participating in some of my personal development sessions and who came to see me for sciatica in her left leg, localized in her left calf. Having already worked with me it was easy for her to quickly come to the realization that she was not accepting something in her life that was trying to be liberated in this way. Her boss, a veritable caricature of the patriarch, had demanded that she change her way of working and had forced her to train someone to help her, whereas for various reasons (and out of certain fears) she was fiercely independent and even solitary. The tension of this inner conflict was released from her calf in one session, but almost immediately it moved to her thigh and hip when she realized that her boss had a hidden agenda: he was angling to replace her with the other person, who seemed to him to be easier to handle. We had to work on freeing up her hip, not only physically, but also in terms of its psychological implications.

When tension manifests in the right calf it is yin-related and expresses the maternal dynamic. Claudine had consulted with me about other problems and came to see me for sciatica in the right leg, concentrated in a line below the knee. I explained to her the possible meaning of this pain while I worked on her body and her energies. Suddenly she began crying quietly and told me about a difficult situation at work. She had to make an important decision about her career under not insignificant pressure from her company (which represents the mother). This decision, however, was very difficult for her to accept because if she left her current position she was going to have to abandon someone she had been protecting, and she feared that this person would suffer a lot if she left.

◆ ◆ ◆

The significance of the lower parts of the body, in the legs, is represented in the following illustration:

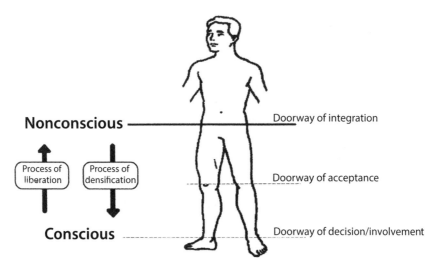

Fig. 4.4. Symbolism of the lower limbs

Anytime we experience tension in the lower limbs it is a sign of tension in our relationships with others (desire, intentions, impossibility, inability, fear, etc.) or in our relationship to ourself that is linked to our own supposed inability or to something from the outside that disables us. We are holding an attitude, a role, or a position in which we cannot *be* or don't know how to *be* or don't manage to *be*.

The Upper Limbs

Attached to the upper body at the level of the shoulders, the upper limbs allow us to touch, grasp, and take. They are also used to reject, surround, hold tightly, smother, or imprison. Essentially the arms allow us to act—they are vehicles of action. By "action" we mean mastery, strength, and power. The arms are what give us the possibility of acting on others and

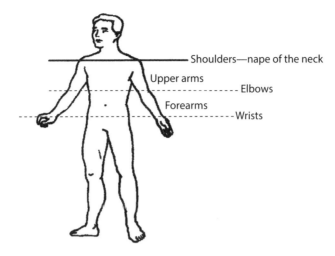

Fig. 4.5. The upper limbs

on things, choosing or judging them. The arms allow us to protect and defend others and ourself. Inasmuch as they are vehicles of action and choice, they facilitate passing from the conceptual to the real, to *doing*. Through their agency, *being* is expressed by *doing* (i.e., the conceptual can move into the real, yang can manifest in the yin). Like the legs, the arms are composed of two parts, the upper arm (the biceps and the humerus) and the forearm (the radius and the ulna). These two segments involve three principal joints: the shoulder, the elbow, and the wrist. The upper limbs terminate in a masterful part of the body: the hand.

Issues in the Upper Limbs

Tension in the arms in the form of pain or trauma speaks to us about difficulties in acting on something or someone, or in doing or choosing something in the inner or outer world. A desire to act, to master or control something or someone that cannot be mastered expresses itself in tension that can, as with the legs, lead all the way up to fracture. Pain in any part of the arms can also mean difficulty moving ideas, projects, or concepts that are dear to our hearts into expression in the real world. The precise point where the tension manifests (in the upper arm, the shoulder, the forearm, the wrist) will provide detailed information as to what we consider to be "preventing" us from acting. Our arms also speak to us about our connection to power and to owning things, and consequently, to our ability to let go of things—or not.

As with the legs, we are going to study first of all the axes of the joints and then afterward the upper arm, the lower arm, and the hand, while reserving a special little section for the nape of the neck.

▸ THE SHOULDERS

The shoulders are to the arms what the hips are to the legs. The shoulder is the basic joint, the anchor point, the primary axis of the arm. It represents the axis of our ability and will in relation to action and mastery. Our shoulders carry the unconscious thread of our connection to action and the will for mastery over the world. The capacity to act and the intentional will belong to the symbolism of the shoulder. Everything that touches our deep desire for action on something or someone will therefore have a direct, somatic relationship with the shoulder. Like the hips, the shoulders are the doorway of integration, the doorway of the nonconscious (as shown in figure 4.5), but here it is in relation to action, whereas with the hips it involves a connection to relationship. It is in this area that there emerges a desire and intention to act, to move toward expression in the real world.

The image of the doorway is noteworthy because the bone that connects the tip of the shoulder to the chest at the sternum is the clavicle, a word that comes from the Latin *clavicula,* meaning "little key." The attachment point of the clavicle to the sternum is located right over the throat chakra, the chakra of self-expression. This is even more notable when we think about the fact that the only means of expression for a person is precisely in *doing,* in action for which the shoulders are the doorway.

Shoulder Issues

The tension that we feel in the shoulders (tip of the shoulder, trapezius, clavicle, scapula) speaks to us about difficulties moving into action. It means that we are encountering the feeling that the brakes are being put on our desire for action, notably in terms of how that action will be accomplished. We feel hindered, not from any lack of ability, but from a lack of assistance, or as a result of external opposition. We think that the outside world (or our own internal censor) is preventing us, not allowing us, not giving us the means or authority to act. Energy that cannot then move into the arms (where it can *do*) gets blocked in the shoulders. Very mental people who think a lot and act little often have very painful trapezius muscles.

If it's the left shoulder the tension is related to yang (paternal) symbolism, and if it's the right shoulder it's a yin-related (maternal) dynamic. Andrea came to see me for significant pain in her right shoulder. She was going through a very difficult period with her daughter, who without much forethought had created a gymnastics and dance center for which she had asked her mother to provide financial support and serve as a guarantor. Unfortunately, lack of planning combined with an economic crunch quickly landed the center in serious difficulties. Andrea, who wanted to recuperate and protect her funds, had for several months wanted her daughter to stop her activities. However, legally there was nothing she could do because she was not the manager of the center. She was also not managing to "act" on her daughter, that is, require her to stop her activities. As a result, Andrea felt blocked, unable to undertake anything because the outer world (business contracts, etc.) was preventing her from acting. Meanwhile, her daughter (the yin dynamic) added to her inability to act on the situation. Everything converged to become expressed as pain in Andrea's right shoulder.

▶ THE ELBOWS

The elbows are to the arms what the knees are to the legs. Like the knee the elbow bends, lets go, or gives way. It gives the arm the possibility of multidirectional mobility, extending the arm to all horizontal and vertical axes except backward—the opposite of the knee, which can only bend backward. Difficulty letting go when faced with a will to act that is rigid will be felt in this joint. The elbow represents the doorway of acceptance in relation to action, as shown in figure 4.6 on page 131. It is also a joint that swings between the conscious and the nonconscious, either in the densification of energies (from the nonconscious to the conscious) or the liberation of energies (from the conscious to the non-conscious). It is in this area that in a deep feeling sense we experience our emotions around or our ideas for action based on our acceptance of them.

Elbow Issues

When the elbow hurts it means that we are having difficulty accepting an experience, a situation. Being in the region of the arm, this tension is connected to action, to *doing*. Something is happening or someone is doing something that we reject or that we have a hard time admitting or can only accept under duress. It can also be something that we are compelled to carry out despite misgivings, or that we would have pre-ferred to do differently or not at all. Tension in the elbow also tells us that some way of acting doesn't quite suit us, upsets our habitual way of doing things, or upsets our beliefs in relation to those actions.

If the pain or trauma manifests in the right elbow it is yin-related and connected to maternal symbolism; if it occurs in the left elbow it is yang-related and connected to paternal symbolism. The example that comes to mind here is Hervé, who came to see me for pain in his shoul-ders and biceps. He confirmed that practically the whole left side of his body was tense and in pain. Having had his left salivary glands operated on shortly after his arrival in France from Algeria twenty years ago, he confessed that he had a tendency since then to bump or hurt the left side of his body. At the time of his visit he was suffering especially in his shoulders, and he told me that the pain had moved down into his elbows, with slightly more pain in the left elbow. Hervé's life had taken a significant turn at the time of the events that led to Algeria's indepen-dence in 1962. He was just a boy at that time when his father was taken away and by the authorities. His father had never been heard of since, and Hervé could only assume that he was dead. A few months after his father's disappearance is when his left salivary glands began to seize up. Despite many treatments, he finally had to undergo surgery. The symbolism was clear: he could not "swallow" what had taken place in his life. While the problem had been surgically corrected, the left side of this body continued to sound the alarm bell, trying to communicate his inner pain. Hervé was of a culture that believed that a man is supposed to be strong and not express his feelings outwardly. He had never accepted what had happened to his father, and he felt vulnerable as a result. He confessed that at present he was confronted with problems and constraints in taking action in his professional environment, and that he was having difficulty accepting that, too. He was feeling a lot of pain in his shoulders, biceps, and elbows, indicating a deeply felt sense of being blocked from acting, with a dominance on the left side that was telling him that his paternal wound had definitely not healed.

▸ THE WRISTS

The wrist is a joint of total mobility. It is linked to the elbow through the forearm and allows the hand, the final vehicle of action, to move on all axes in space. It is by means of the wrist that the hand attaches to the arm, giving the hand all possible range of motion. It is the wrist that makes the connection between what is transmitting the action (the arm) and what is carrying out the action (the hand). The wrist represents the doorway of choice, the doorway of involvement, as seen in figure 4.6 on page 131. In this regard it is much like the ankle, but in the case of the elbow the symbolism reflects the world of action. In carrying out an action the arm is the first vehicle, the vehicle of transmission, while the hand is final vehicle, the one of execution. The wrist is the link between the two by giving the hand total mobility, a flexibility and directional precision that it could not otherwise have. The wrist then is what allows movement and flexibility in our actions and opinions. It is the projection of these same qualities in relation to our will and our search for power over things and beings. It is the conscious articulation of our own guidelines for action and of mastery and for the expression of will, whereas the shoulder represents the unconscious articulation of these same guidelines.

Wrist Issues

Sprains, pain, or trauma in the wrists speak to us about our tensions, our lack of flexibility or confidence in our actions or in our desire to act, or in our opinions. This means that our connection to action, to what we do, lacks confidence or stability. As a result we harden our wrists to try to make them more solid. This applies to our search for control over the world (objects, matter, or beings) and over ourself. When we prevent ourself from doing, when we don't give ourself the possibility of doing, our wrists (and consequently our hands) are going to tense up and hurt. We bind the wrists of prisoners when we want to prevent them from acting (whereas it is the feet we bind when we want to prevent them from fleeing). Similarly, when we are willful or excessively authoritarian and the action is happening only from force of will, our wrists will manifest their opposition and calm this excessive willfulness and the use of force by hurting. This is how our inner master obliges us to calm down!

If the pain, trauma, or tension manifests in right wrist, it relates to yin and carries maternal symbolism; if in the left wrist it relates to yang and carries paternal symbolism. This is what happened to me several years ago, after I had been practicing aikido for three years. With my very willful nature I had a noticeable tendency in my practice to want to force things, to reproduce in physical form the same type of mental connection I had with life. It was clear that my assiduous aikido practice was giving me more and more personal power over the external world. The risk was that this power, when combined with my strong will, was going to produce an unintentionally dangerous combination because it was a power that I had not yet completely mastered. My inner master must have been watching out for me because during one aikido training workshop my wrists became more and more painful every day, to the point where I could no longer hold my partner in the exercises. I didn't have any choice—I had to let go and release my grip, my way of holding the world, and in this case it involved the way I held my partners in aikido practice. I did not understand the message right away and was very troubled by this very unfair handicap, against which I rebelled. For two years I bandaged my wrists before aikido practice, and in my professional work I had to take my wrist pain into account while I was working. However, the pain eventually forced me to change my attitude and way of working. One day I finally came to understand the extent to which my relationship with the world had been thought-based and willful. From that day on I no longer had trouble with my wrists, even though I use them all day long and sometimes very intensively (in seminars, training sessions, client sessions, massages, and so forth).

▸ THE HANDS

The hand is the masterful part of the arm, much the way the foot is to the leg. The hands represent the final stage by which all acts are carried out, including all the fine details. The word *manual,* "of, relating to, or involving the hands," has the same root as the word *manifestation.* Since the hand represents moving from the conceptual to the real, from the theoretical to the practical, it is also an instrument for speaking and communicating. This is true not only for those who are deaf, but for many different cultures where hand gestures are often more powerful and revealing than words.

Many studies have demonstrated the importance of nonverbal communication. This is the first form of communication that we experience and experiment with in life. In the relationship between a mother and a child the exchange of signs of recognition and affection are made by means of touch, with the hands. The hands are therefore vehicles of transmission and communication. They both give and receive. They can also serve as sense organs, with touch and feeling oftentimes replacing the eyes as vehicles of perception. It is with the hands that we perceive or transmit energy. The laying on of hands is a spiritual, therapeutic, and calming gesture. The palm and each of the fingers are emitters and captors of our energies. An acupuncture meridian begins or ends in each one of the fingers, as described in the section that follows on the fingers. The particular meridian in each finger determines which type of energy is being transmitted. We will look into this in a moment when we study each finger.

Inasmuch as the hand is an implement of execution, of acting, it is also a vector of power and strength. In many cultures the hand represents royal power and even divine power (as in something being "in the hands of God"). The hand allows us to grasp, hold, imprison, and crush. The way people shake hands is indicative of how they envision the relationship they have with the person they are greeting. When two people hold hands they abandon their desire to have any power over the other and in fact join with each other in affection.

For the most part the role of the hand corresponds to that of the arm; the difference is that the hand acts in the final stage, while the arm transmits. We can symbolically compare the whole arm to an arrow, with the hand representing the tip, whereas the arm is the shaft. The movement of the arrow is transmitted by the shaft (the arm), but it is the tip (the hand) that ensures penetration into the target.

Issues in the Hand

Hand issues speak to our connection to action in the external world. Tension, pain, or trauma in the hands means that our connection to this world is one of mastery, control, possessiveness, or greed. It means that we are being excessive in wanting to hold on to or control things or people, either through force of will in a desire to dominate, or out of fear. The hand that closes up is a hand that fears that things or people are going to escape it, and the hand that closes up in a fist wants to strike out at something or someone.

As I sometimes explain to clients, life and everything that happens in it can be symbolized by a handful of sand. If we want to have it and keep it, we have to keep the hand open because if we close it the sand will escape through the cracks. The hand that is peaceful or welcoming is always open, whereas the hand that struggles, that cries out for vengeance or that threatens is always closed. Hands and wrists are closely linked, and pain in this area usually affects both, indicating a lot of trouble in letting go of the world, that is, in letting go of will, mastery, possession, or power over the world.

Dominique, age forty, was suffering from **rheumatoid arthritis,** a condition for which she had already undergone multiple surgeries. Generous and passionate, she had a connection with the world that was one of very developed yet unconscious power. In continuous struggle with life and people, she decreed and directed everything in her life in a very unaware way. Her natural generosity facilitated this, yet those around her were forced to adjust, each in their own way, to her character and attitude. She chose a husband who was physically strong and powerful, yet weak and uncertain in relation to his own will to act decisively. Dominique therefore found that she was the one who was always obliged to act, to do, to direct, to exercise her will for him because, she thought, "He's not able." Her relationship to power, however, was out of balance, and had manifested in a form of rheumatism that afflicted her in both of her hands and wrists. Notably, the form of rheumatism Dominique suffered from is regarded as being progressive. No one knows how to stop it (i.e., *no one can have power over it*). It is also considered an autoimmune disorder, which means it is a disorder in which the organism destroys itself because it no longer recognizes certain of its own cells and in fact perceives them as "enemy" cells. Why would Dominique's body believe that the cells of her wrists and hands are her enemies? Could it be that her hands and wrists, as vehicles of action, of doing, were being misused in terms of her distorted sense of power, and that she wasn't using them in a way that supported her life, her stability, her happiness, and the realization of her Life Path? The key for Dominique was to help her to understand the source of her pain. Her misuse of power had to be put in a different light so that she would be able to try to change her behavior. Through our work together I believe

Dominique received everything she needed to help her think deeply about her condition, and not a moment too soon, as other parts of her body were beginning to be affected by the disease, while her wrists and hands had already been operated on numerous times.

▶ THE FINGERS

Fingers represent the fine end points of the hands. They are the "details" of the hands and consequently the final endings of our actions, the details of how we act. Each finger represents a specific detail, mode, or phase that can be deciphered based on which energetic meridian ends or begins in the finger, and so these meridians provide us with important feedback. Because each one of the fingers has a specific energetic point at the tip, we can stimulate or clear unconsciously but effectively any possible tensions to be found there.

Because of the energetic points at the tip of each finger, the fingers are favored locations for multiple daily mishaps that appear to be meaningless and ruled by chance. But it is never by chance that we cut, jam, burn, crush, or twist a certain finger. In every case there is a precise process taking place that seeks to express or clear a tension. This process is reliable because the energetic point at the tip of each finger is also a "source point" or "springtime point," indicating a possible rebirth of energy with the release of tension, thanks to which a new dynamic can appear or through which the old dynamic can "reconnect to source" and change polarity.

Finger Issues

This section gives the overall meaning of each of the fingers and the meaning of the injuries that each finger will express. The energetic meridians that terminate or begin at the end of each finger impart their dynamics to the fingers and explain the deeper meaning of the tensions that appear in each finger. Bear in mind that if any form of tension manifests in a finger of the right hand it is related to yin (maternal) symbolism, and if it manifests in a finger of the left hand it is connected to yang (paternal) symbolism.

The thumb: The thumb is the finger where the Lung meridian ends. It is the finger of protection, defense, and reactivity in relation to the external world. The thumbs-up and thumbs-down sign is a universally recognized form of nonverbal communication. Among young children all over the world **thumb-sucking** is a means of reassurance. I find it interesting that nowadays more and more young children have been sucking their middle finger or ring finger instead of the thumb, which is no doubt indicative of a shift in orientation as regards security, as the thumb represents external security, protection through defense, whereas the middle and ring fingers represent the search for security not through defense, but through unity. This need for inner and outer (oneself and the family) unity is associated with a search for power, for action on the external world. The thumb can also represent sadness or defeat. In all cases trauma (cuts, sprains, burns) or pathologies of the thumb (**rheumatism, arthrosis**) are related to the need for protection or defense against an aggression coming from the external world, whether imaginary or real, or possibly to an experience of defeat or sadness.

The index finger: This is the finger where the Large Intestine meridian begins. It is a finger of protection, but in the sense of clearing things or tossing them out. This means it is the finger of demand, of authority, of accusation, or even of threat. The index finger orders, directs, and indicates which direction is threatening. Pain that manifest in this finger is related to a need to clear something from oneself that is unacceptable and needs to be eliminated, including anything threatening. Most of time it's a matter of simply clearing an experience to which we haven't agreed. Issues in the index finger can also express an excessive tendency to be bossy or authoritarian, a dynamic that needs to be cleared because it is excessive.

The middle finger: This is the finger where the Heart Protector meridian terminates. It is the finger of inner structuring, of the inner government of things, and also the finger of sexuality (a form of power over others that brings pleasure). It represents satisfaction with our experience and with the action that we have on the world. Tensions that manifest in it speak to us about the dissatisfaction that we have about the way things happen or the way we manage those things in life.

The ring finger: This is the finger where the Triple Heater meridian begins. It represents the union of things, their cohesion and their assimilation within us. It carries the ring of marriage or union, whatever its form might be. Its trauma or pathology speaks to us about difficulties in uniting with things in us or around us. Pain here tells us about difficulties in creating coherence among all the different aspects of the self to find meaning.

The little finger: This is the only finger that has two meridians side by side. They are the Heart meridian (which terminates here) and the Small Intestine meridian (which begins here). The little finger is the finger of finesse, of what is elaborated, but also of what is emotional and superficial; it is the finger of appearances or pretensions. This is the finger we raise when we drink tea in a "high-society" way, giving elegance to our gesture. Tension in this finger indicates a need to externalize either an inner tension of an emotional order or a tendency to superficiality or subjectivity. We may be too invested in the role we play in society or too caught up in appearances and not interested enough in the natural, in simply being.

▸ THE UPPER ARM (BICEPS AND HUMERUS)

Recall that the shoulder and the shoulder blades are the unconscious representation of the nonconscious relationship to action. They represent the point of emergence or resurgence of the nonconscious in its connection to action in the world and on beings (including ourself), which I term the doorway of integration. As for the elbow, it is the demarcation line of acceptance. The upper arm, built around the humerus, the long bone of the upper arm, is located between the shoulder and the elbow and links them. It therefore represents the movement of wishes and desires for action from the nonconscious to the conscious. With the upper arm we are in a process of densification at the moment preceding conscious acceptance. The upper arm can also act from the conscious to the nonconscious, a direction indicative of a process of liberation at the moment that follows conscious acceptance of those wishes and desires (see figure 4.6 on page 131).

Issues in the Upper Arm

Tension in the upper arms (sore spots, cramps, brachial neuralgia, etc.) is the manifestation of difficulties acting on what we feel. In a person's relationship with his ability to act, the deep, unconscious wounds or memories that come to the surface, which he refuses to accept, will manifest as pain in the upper arm. This can be as extreme as a fracture of the humerus if the memory that surfaces is too strong and disturbing to the structure (the bone) of personal beliefs or life choices of the person. Personal failure, the impossibility of carrying out something professionally or within the family, or fears in relation to an action or its consequences will be expressed, if need be, through pain or trauma in the upper arms. It can be a matter of actions that have already been experienced that the person has accepted consciously but that he cannot or is not yet ready to accept in the depths of himself. This can be true for someone who has to give up something that he considered important for himself (a project, a promotion, etc.), a decision he understands and accepts, but in his depths he cannot accept. Despite all the logical reasons that have allowed him to understand things he refuses or cannot integrate on a deeper level. If the pain or trauma is located in the humerus it means that the tension is linked to a deep structure, to the unconscious beliefs and values of the person in relation to his actions. If, on the other hand, it manifests in the muscles, we are faced with a manifestation that is less serious because it is less anchored in the structure.

When pain or a fracture occurs in the right arm it is related to yin, maternal symbolism. If the pain or fracture happens in the left arm, it is related to yang, paternal symbolism. Let's return to the example of Hervé whom I mentioned earlier in the discussion of the elbow (see page 118). The tension he was experiencing in his work environment was being expressed clearly in his arms, shoulders, and elbows. Hervé felt he couldn't act or that things were not happening as he wished because of the external world (as indicated by the pain in his shoulders). Unconsciously he knew and understood the reasons (arms) for that, but he had difficulty accepting those reasons or even simply noticing (elbows) them—no doubt because he felt the situation he was in was unfair. As a result, the energy remained stuck in his upper arms.

▶ THE FOREARM, THE RADIUS, AND THE ULNA

The radius and the ulna lie between the elbow and the wrist. We have seen that the elbow represents the demarcation line of acceptance, and that the wrist is the demarcation line of involvement in the sense of choice (and not of decision, as with the ankle). The forearm is the first stage of moving through the will to act in the world of accomplishments. When we want to do something, something that touches our deep memories (the nonconscious), and we accept it (elbow), we must then choose and do what will allow us to carry it out. If doing that is difficult because, for example, we have difficulty deciding on the means, we are going to develop tension in the form of pain or cramps in the forearm, or even fracture the ulna and/or radius bones if the tension is severe enough.

This is the part of the body that precedes or follows the hand and the wrist depending on which direction the energies are circulating (whether densification or liberation). It can involve moving things from the nonconscious to the conscious (elbow to hand), in which case it is a process of densification at the moment that follows conscious acceptance, which precedes the movement into the real (wrist, hand) through doing. But it can also involve moving things from the conscious to the nonconscious (hand to elbow), in which case it is a process of liberation at the moment that precedes nonconscious acceptance, which follows movement into the real.

Issues in the Forearm, Ulna, and Radius

Problems in these areas of the body speak to us about difficulties accepting actions or doings that we encounter in life. Difficulty in choosing to act or in giving ourself the means to act (means that may be new or different from the usual way we act), or difficulty in finding certainty in our actions can manifest as pain in this area of the arm. A fracture can occur in one or both bones of the upper arm when the inner tension is too strong or when our blockages in relation to the action or choice are so anchored, rigidified, or fossilized that they cannot admit the torsion (obligation to change) imposed from the outside. Then it is the ulna or radius or both that finally give way. Simple stiffness in the forearm means that we are having difficulty budging, in giving the wrist or the hand free play. If the tension manifests in the left forearm it is yang-related (father symbolism), and if it manifests in right forearm it is yin-related (mother symbolism).

The Neck

The neck connects the brain and its "doers," the arms and legs. Originating from the cervical plexus, which is located at the base of the neck, all desires and decisions to act are sent in the direction of the organ or limb that is best suited to carry them out. The neck is therefore the place where desires and intentions have not yet emerged, have not yet begun to appear, and have not yet led to initiating a physical movement. Such impulses have not yet been connected to the outside. The neck therefore represents the transit point from the conceptual mode (brain, ideas, concepts, desires, intentions, etc.) to the action mode (executing, relating, expressing, etc.).

Issues in the Neck

Tension, pain, or blockages in the neck usually occur in the nape, or back, of the neck. They speak about difficulties moving into the real world with our desires, ideas, concepts, and wishes. However, in contrast to tension in the shoulders, which generally means the same thing, in the case of the nape of the neck we are at the stage where things have not arrived "at the doorway" of moving into action. This means that we cannot move them into the real world because we think we are not able to. Not being able to is due to our own inner belief, whereas in the case of blockage in the shoulders the inability is imposed by others, by the external world. If the discomfort in the neck spreads to one of the shoulders, this will provide supplementary information as to yin or yang symbolism (in terms of why we think we are not able).

The simplest example I can offer is that of **torticollis** (a stiff neck). This kind of tension can prevent us, sometimes painfully so, from turning the head to the right or the left. And what is the universal meaning of this movement of turning the head right and left? In all cultures of the world this movement means "no." It is a sign of disagreement, refusal, or nonacceptance of what is happening or of what someone else says or does. A stiff neck prevents us from making this gesture. It means our inability to say no to someone or to a situation. We think we don't have the right or the ability to refuse.

Bernard was a senior manager in a very large French distribution company who attended one of my corporate seminars on the dynamic of relationships. For three days this man had been suffering from a very stiff neck. I asked him if he was experiencing a situation in which he wanted to say no but couldn't because he thought he couldn't or didn't have the right to. At first disconcerted by my question, he nevertheless thought about it for a few moments and then suddenly, to his own stupefaction, he recognized that indeed he was experiencing a professional situation of just this type. The CEO of his group, of which Bernard was one of the principal regional representatives, had a mania for organizing prestige meetings for his staff that Bernard termed "a High Mass."

These meetings, which lasted from one to three days, didn't accomplish much in Bernard's opinion except to make him lose time when he had lots to do in the field. It was impossible for him to refuse to attend these meetings, he said, because he risked displeasing his boss, who might then see him in a bad light. He had just learned three days before my seminar that yet another one of his boss's meetings was going to take place the following month, which was when he had planned to visit the regional stores he was in charge of. Bernard had learned the news of this meeting Monday evening, and Tuesday morning he woke up with a neck so stiff that he still couldn't move his head by Thursday, the day of my seminar. He decided then and there to think about how he could express his disagreement with his boss or else he would have to find some way to accept the "High Masses."

The major axes of the upper limbs—arms, shoulders, and the nape of the neck—are summarized in the figure below, which shows what is happening and how.

Anytime we experience tension in the upper part of the body it is a sign that in our connection to action (desire, will, impossibility,

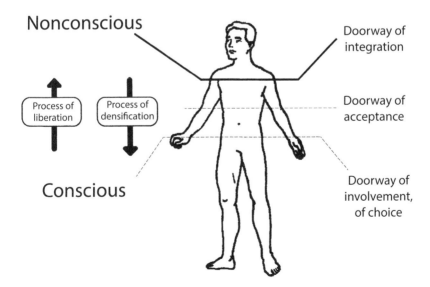

Fig. 4.6. Symbolism of the upper limbs

inability, fear, etc.) or to power over things and beings, we are experiencing an equivalent tension linked either to our supposed inability to act (nape of the neck), or to an inability coming from the exterior (shoulder). We are confronting something that we cannot, don't know how to, or cannot manage to *do*.

The Trunk

The trunk is the central part of the body to which the limbs attach permitting it to move around and act. It is also the part in which are found all the organs that ensure supply management. The trunk represents the individual's house in which are gathered all the "functional" organs, the "decisional" organ (the brain) being placed above it. It constitutes the axis of the body, the central engine that produces and distributes energy. Human alchemy takes place in it. Like the trunk of a tree, it is the most imposing part but the least mobile and the least supple. It contains all the functional organs and the spinal column. It is through the organs—that is, through the twelve energetic organ meridians— that the trunk engages in expressing itself, allowing possible tensions to manifest as physical or psychological symptoms. In the next chapter we will go through the body's main organ systems—digestive, respiratory, urinary, circulatory, nervous, and reproductive—to connect the role of each organ to its psychological representation.

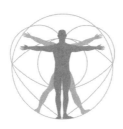

5

The Major Systems
of the Body

The Symbolism of Our Organ Systems

When we stumble, it is not the foot that is to blame.

Chinese proverb

A biological system is a complex network of biologically relevant entities. Different body systems consist of collections of cells, tissues, and organs with a common purpose. Each system has a well-defined function and is part of a whole, integrated system. There is the digestive system, the respiratory system, the urinary system, the circulatory system, the nervous system, and the reproductive system. First, we will look at each system and its role. Then we will go into details about the organs involved, not from a medical point of view because that is not our aim, but to simply show the function fulfilled by each system and the meaning of issues that affect it. It is necessary for the better understanding of each organ system to refer to its energetic representation—its meridian and which one of the Five Principles it expresses. In this way we will connect the organ system to its psychoenergetic environment.

The Digestive System

The digestive system allows us to digest solid and liquid food. It is thanks to this system that we can assimilate the material nourishment that the earth offers us and that good cooking refines for our pleasure. By means of an extremely developed alchemy the digestive system makes food usable and acceptable to our organism, to ultimately become our final fuel—energy. The digestive system contains the most organs of any other system in the body. This helps us understand how extensive and elaborate its alchemy is, as solid food is a denser form of energy that must be transformed; therefore multiple operations are needed. That is why before being able to move into the blood, nutritional substances must first make their way through a number of receptacles and receive a certain number of additives (for example, the stomach must produce hydrochloric acid) to dissolve them. The digestive system is composed of the mouth, the esophagus, the stomach, the liver, the gallbladder, the spleen, the pancreas, the small intestine, and the large intestine. Since the mouth has an important role and a very particular signification, I will specifically come back to it on page 169.

Issues in the Digestive System

Issues in the digestive system tell us about our difficulty swallowing, digesting, or assimilating what is taking place in life. "I couldn't swallow what he told me" or "I still haven't digested what you said" or "That stayed in the pit of my stomach" are some popular expressions that invoke the role of the digestive system. Based on the specific digestive organ involved we can bring some precision to tension or difficulties we are experiencing there.

▶ THE STOMACH

The stomach is the organ that first receives through the esophagus the unprocessed food that has been prepared by chewing. It is therefore the first receptacle of material nourishment. The stomach has a big job—it plays the role of cement mixer, mixing and blending, but also dissolving ingested food thanks to hydrochloric acid, thereby preparing it for assimilation. The stomach is therefore in charge of the directly material side of digestion. It must take charge of and master food's materiality.

Stomach Issues

Stomach issues speak to us about difficulties or tension we encounter in our effort to master or manage the material world. Financial, professional, scholarly, or legal setbacks will choose to be expressed in this way if they stimulate real or imaginary worry in us. Given its role in the mixing of food, the stomach's making us suffer can also mean that we have a tendency to ruminate, to go over and over things and events in an obsessive way. That's when gastric acidity can tell us to stop.

Stomach ulcers are often the result of professional setbacks, and for a long time they were the "preferred" illness of successful businessmen. The numbers have decreased nowadays because we now know how to silence the stomach. The many students who have felt cramps or acidity in the stomach before exams know to what an extent they are a sign of anxiety. **Acidity, acid reflux, ulcers,** or **stomach cancer** are all manifestations of progressive intensity that express difficulties in digesting what we are experiencing, while vomiting is a sign of pure and simple rejection, out-and-out refusal to accept shocks from life or situations that do not satisfy us.

▶ THE SPLEEN AND PANCREAS

These two organs participate in digestion; the pancreas is involved in producing secretions that discharge into the small intestine, while the spleen handles the composition of blood through the manufacture and storage of red and white blood cells. The pancreas controls, through the insulin that it manufactures, the level of sugar that we have in the blood, and along with the pancreatic juices it participates actively in the digestion of food prepared by the stomach. These two organs express the Earth element; they are plodding, field-worker-type organs that mainly concentrate on digestive duties.

Issues in the Spleen and Pancreas

Problems here mean that there is a tendency to move through life too reasonably, that is, without leaving enough room for pleasure, for joy. Duty is important since professional and material accomplishment requires it, but life can be lacking in gentleness and playfulness, which we all need. Material worries held inside and obsessive anxiety, fear of missing out or of not knowing or not being up to something can manifest as problems in the spleen or pancreas. The tendency to live in the past for fear of not being able to manage the present, or cultivating memories of the past can manifest as tension or illness in these organs. The overarching need to conform to norms, to respect the rules, is often expressed through upsets in the spleen or pancreas. This is reflected at the energetic level because it is the energy of the spleen/pancreas that, among other things, is in charge of the monthly menstrual cycle.* As well, those who suffer from **diabetes,** a condition of the pancreas, must be very vigilant about regularity in their lives. The timing of meals and all of life's routines must be perfectly regulated and respected as scrupulously as possible so as not to set off an attack.

Pancreatic upsets can take two forms: **hypoglycemia** (a lack of sugar in the blood) and **hyperglycemia** or diabetes (excess sugar in the blood). What does sugar represent? It is sweetness, kindness, and, by extension, it is a proof of love or recognition. In all the cultures of the world something sweet is the gift given to children when they've been good (respected the rules), when they've had good marks at school (responded to societal norms), or simply when we want to give them pleasure (a maternal gesture). Excess sugar in the blood expresses that we are having difficulty managing, experiencing, or getting sweetness in our lives. Diabetes frequently means that the person

---

*Translator's note: Notably, the French word for "menstrual period" also means "rules."

had a father who was excessively and often unfairly authoritarian (an excess of rules and norms) and that the person found refuge in the protective sweetness of the mother. Food (the mother) then becomes a significant palliative, which can lead to progressive and inexorable weight gain.

Certain strong psychological shocks in which the person is confronted with the brutal destruction of emotional securities or beliefs can be expressed by the onset of diabetes. I am thinking here about a young woman named Daniele who came to see me because she wanted to have a child but her diabetes prevented it. Analysis of her situation allowed us to return to a tragic event that occurred in her childhood. When she was about age seven she was walking one day on the side of a road with her sister. A car coming from the opposite direction veered toward them for no reason and hit her little sister, whom she adored. With unmitigated terror she saw her sister die before her very eyes. For several weeks she was unable to speak about or express her suffering over the loss of what was most dear to her and filled her life with sweetness and joy. Six months later, the first signs of diabetes appeared in the girl. After three sessions working on this emotional memory and on the energies concerned, Daniele's sugar levels began to decrease slowly but steadily. In conjunction with this work I advised her to consult a friend who is a homeopathic doctor so that our work would be accompanied by medical assistance designed to stimulate the pancreatic functions and not replace them. But lest I forget the most important thing: a few months later Daniele gave birth to a daughter.

Hypoglycemia (a lack of sugar) speaks about a reverse form of suffering linked to the inability or difficulty in receiving, accepting, or thinking we have the right to sweetness. This is common in children who are not wanted by their mother and/or for whom the father is absent. The absence of maternal refuge produces negative associations with food so that one does not like it or even accept it (as in the case of anorexia), or that one assimilates it only when there's no choice but to do so, so that assimilating food happens without pleasure and without sweetness. The search for missing norms or rules makes for an angular and emaciated physique in which the roundness (sweetness) is missing.

▶ THE LIVER

The liver is a highly developed and versatile organ. It is the biggest organ in the human body. It plays an essential role in digestion through the secretion of bile, but it also ensures another very important activity, the filtering of the blood. It thus participates in the composition of blood and its quality just as much at a nutritional level as at an immune-system level (defense, healing, storing). The liver gives to the blood its texture, its composition, its vibration, its coloration. Its double role is reflected in the fact that it receives a double blood supply: one from the hepatic artery that provides it with oxygen, and the other from the hepatic portal vein that carries nutrients to it assimilated by the small intestine. These two channels meet in the liver, coming together in the inferior vena cava. This latter conduit transports the blood that is enriched with nutrients and other globules, then redistributes it throughout the body thanks to the heart after having been enriched with oxygen by the lungs.

Issues with the Liver

Liver problems are a sign that it is hard for us to digest something in life, but these issues are more finely nuanced than stomach issues. The main emotion associated with the liver is anger. Tension and discomfort in this organ can mean that our habitual and excessive mode of reacting to life's demands is anger. Every time we handle problems with the external world by yelling and getting angry we are mobilizing all the energy of the liver in that direction, thereby depriving it each time of a large part of the energy it needs to function. The liver will manifest this imbalance by not correctly playing its role in the digestive phase. Conversely, anger that is too often suppressed will make the energy of the liver more dense, thereby risking a more significant pathology such as cirrhosis, cysts, or cancer.

Liver issues also speak to us about difficulties in experiencing or accepting our sentiments, our emotions, or those that others send our way. The image we have of ourself or the image that others give us of ourself depends to a great extent on the liver. This determines our enjoyment of life, which is what we find in the liver's job of filtering and nourishing the blood. Tension in the liver can mean that our image has been brought into question through our experience, and that our enjoyment of life has been taken over by bitterness and inner acidity toward the external world which does not give us the recognition and respect we expect. Guilt—a liver quality—obliges us to justify ourself, to defend ourself.

The liver participates intensively in immune-system functioning by helping us develop our acquired immunity based on experiences undergone by the organism. Liver energy mobilizes our psychological defenses and often our anger. If this occurs frequently it weakens the energy of the liver and then the gallbladder, to which it is connected. The liver is a yin organ that represents feelings that have to do with our deeper being (while the gallbladder, which is yang, is connected to our social being).

▸ THE GALLBLADDER

The gallbladder works directly with the liver, from which it gathers and concentrates bile. It then redistributes it into the small intestine, right at the exit point of the stomach. The release of bile allows the digestive process, notably the fatty elements, to proceed in a harmonious way. In the case of malfunction, digestion is perceived as being "bad."

Issues in the Gallbladder

As the gallbladder is intrinsic to the physical digestive process, it plays an equivalent role in the psychological digestion of events. Issues in the gallbladder speak of difficulty in clarifying and managing our emotions. One of the definitions of the word *bilious* says as much: "of or indicative of a peevish, ill-natured disposition." And an everyday

French expression that people use when someone is worried translates as "you're making bile." But such worries are always linked to someone (ourselves or someone else) who is dear to us. This emotional response is a yang dynamic, one connected to external events and people. "What is my place?" "Am I acknowledged by others?" "Am I loved for what I do and represent?" Such are the questions about which tension in the gallbladder speaks to us, as well as the violent anger that accompanies difficult junctures, especially when the person feels that something is unjust. Justifying one's actions is also an aspect of this energy, all the more so if a person's actions are not founded in sincerity and truth. Issues with the gallbladder can in fact mean that our sense of the true and the just is not clear or is excessive; they can also mean that we have a tendency to constrain or use or even manipulate others (always, of course, giving ourself good reasons for doing so).

▶ THE SMALL INTESTINE

The small intestine is about twenty feet long. This allows it a large surface area that is augmented by innumerable little inner bumps and crevasses, all of which support the digestive metabolism that finishes the final transformation of nutritional elements before they pass into the blood. The sorting-out of what can be assimilated from what cannot continues then in the large intestine. Everything that can be assimilated goes into the blood and the lymphatic system.

It is important to know that the small intestine is not simply a filter that either lets food pass or not; it participates actively in digestion by secreting essential enzymes, and it also plays an important role in the transport of certain sugars and amino acids. It is therefore through the small intestine that the final selection among the elements moving through it takes place.

Issues in the Small Intestine

Diarrhea and **ulcers,** two of the more common problems involving the small intestine, speak to us about our difficulties in assimilating experiences, in letting them penetrate us without judging them. This organ acts as a kind of customs officer, allowing one particular piece of information through or rejecting some other piece. The small intestine is the physical representative of subjectivity, of reality as it is perceived rather than as it exists independent of one's personal attitudes and perceptions. Pain or sickness in the small intestine can also mean that we have too much of a tendency to judge events and other people, to reason excessively in terms of good and bad, right and wrong. The astrological sign of Virgo, which is very much shaped around concepts of values, around their precision and respect for them, is a good example of this organ. Not surprisingly, many Virgo natives tend toward intestinal fragility.

▶ THE LARGE INTESTINE

The large intestine is the garbage man or clearing agent of the body. It transports and supports the elimination of organic materials that we have ingested that have not been assimilated. This is how the organism avoids getting blocked up, clogged, saturated, and consequently poisoned with matter it cannot handle. Just think of the important role that garbage collectors play in big cities, especially when there is a garbage collectors' strike. This organ also contributes to the proper "breathing" of the body as evacuation of toxic waste from the body makes respiration easier. This explains why in energy work the Large Intestine meridian is the complement of the Lung meridian.

Issues in the Large Intestine

Tension in the form of pain in the large intestine means that we are holding on to things, that we are not letting them depart. Fear of missing out, of being mistaken, excessive holding back (timidity), or refusing to abandon or let go are expressed as problems in the large intestine such as **constipation, bloating, gas,** and so forth. These troubles speak to us also of our difficulty in self-healing, as in forgiving and releasing bad experiences. Excessive acidity often indicates the added presence of an anger that has been suppressed. Just as this organ allows us to eliminate and reject what we have ingested (food) that we cannot assimilate, it also allows us to reject and clear experiences that we have lived through (ingested) that we haven't accepted.

The Respiratory System

The respiratory system allows us to breathe as its name indicates. Thanks to it we can assimilate energy from the air. However, its function is much more extensive than we might think and is not limited to breathing the ambient air. The respiratory system includes the lungs, of course, but also the skin and all the cells of the body. There are in fact two distinct levels of respiration: the breathing called *external,* and the breathing called *internal.* External breathing is the one we know about, that is, pulmonary respiration. But there is another form of external breathing called *cutaneous,* referring to the skin, which plays a large role in respiration. This form of external breathing is that of gas exchanges of oxygen and carbon dioxide through the skin. Internal breathing is respiration that happens at the cellular level, where intracellular changes take place directly. The cells themselves enter into certain gaseous exchanges that are not due to the classic contribution made by the blood. The same process exists at the energetic level.

As an organ attached to the respiratory system, the skin also plays the role of protecting the body in its contact with the external world. As a supple but effective envelope, it protects the body from most aggression, whether it is due to active agents (microbes, viruses, insects, etc.) or passive agents (dust, temperature, rain, etc.). As an essential sensor it also plays an important role in the protective management of external stimuli and demands and in the healing of wounds.

Issues in the Respiratory System

The respiratory system belongs to the element Metal, whose main function is protection in relation to the external world. This protection comes in two forms: filtering dust and gaseous exchanges (rejecting carbon dioxide), and responding to environmental aggression (toxicity). Another of its essential functions is that of healing, the closing up of wounds.

Problems in the respiratory system speak to us of difficulty protecting ourself against the external world, in finding adaptive responses when faced with real or imaginary threats. Respiratory problems may also mean that we're not managing to close or we don't want to close certain wounds in our life, in which case the problems may be speaking to us of sadness, grudges, resentments, and difficulty or refusal to forgive and forget, to let go of a desire to settle scores or worse still, of a desire to take vengeance.

▶ THE LUNGS

The lungs are the principal organs of breathing. It is here that the fundamental exchange of oxygen and carbon dioxide is carried out, without which we would be unable to live. This process happens in minute pockets called *alveoli,* tiny sacs of which we have about 300 million. These sacs are profusely irrigated by means of capillaries that allow the blood (specifically red blood cells) to release the carbon dioxide they contain and recharge themselves with oxygen that will go on to feed all the cells. The membranes of these alveoli are permeable to permit this exchange. If these membranes were spread out flat, you would have a surface of several hundred square yards.

You can imagine how fragile the tissue of these membranes are and the damage caused by the polluted air we breathe, notably from cigarette smoking. Moreover, the lungs are the only natural orifices that are permanently open to the outside and that must constantly be up to defending themselves and defending us. A whole system exists in playing this role. In the passage of air through the nose it is warmed and partially filtered by nose hairs and humidified by the mucus there, which captures some of the dust before it penetrates the bronchi. There the mucus retains the last particles of dust, which are expelled by coughing or by vibrating cilia that sweep them upward.

We can appreciate the extent of this system of protection and defense. In the digestive system there is a process of "destructuring" food that is very sophisticated, whereas in the lungs it is a process of protection. Breathing is the only automatic (unconscious and involuntary) organic function that we can also affect consciously. It is managed by the central autonomic nervous system, but we can nevertheless change our breathing patterns intentionally with the support of the central nervous system. This helps us more easily understand the reason why relaxation techniques using breathing are so effective—because they promote the calming of the autonomic nervous system and as a result, the release of unconsciously held tension.

Issues in the Lungs

Weakness or illness in the lungs expresses a difficulty managing situations with the external world. The simplest example is that of temperatures dropping at the beginning of winter. Those who don't respond by rebalancing their internal thermal system are going to catch cold—the weakened pulmonary system opens the door to flu or a cold. **Coughing, asthma, sore throat,** and **bronchitis** are typical signs that we are feeling a significant pull from the outside world, or perhaps even an aggression, and that we don't know how to manage it (although illness in the lungs is the body's way of clearing this kind of tension). A dry, hacking cough shows that the aggression is irritating and hard to put up with, causing us to react violently. Phlegmy coughs are a sign that the agents of aggression remain imprisoned within us. They are glued to the bronchial mucus that we have to secrete in greater and greater quantities to spit up or clear what is aggressing us and sticking to us.

When I was a teenager I was a rather timid kid, although readily enthusiastic (to hide my timidity). Thin even though a big eater, I had weak lungs and for many years had chronic bronchitis that the family doctor tried to kill with antibiotics. Fortunately, I was living in the country, and country traditions plus the natural common sense of my parents meant that the most often used therapy—as well as the most effective—was the use of cupping glasses and poultices. Each setback or difficulty that I went through at that time was converted into coughing fits first, then developed into flu or bronchitis. To improve upon all of that, at sixteen I began smoking. It was only upon changing my relationship to life and to other people, where I stopped trying to compete with the world, that my pulmonary weakness disappeared and that, as chance would have it, I no longer needed or even wanted to smoke. And that's how it still is today.

The relationship of breathing to how one relates to others can be found in homeopathy with the use of the homeopathic remedy GELSEMIUM. Without going into too much detail, this remedy is prescribed to people who suffer from timidity or from anticipatory fear (such as fear before exams), but it is also very effective for complications of flu and other pulmonary infections. GELSEMIUM is not the only homeopathic remedy that shows us to what an extent homeopathy and energy function at the same level and according to the same laws.

The experience of aggression does not have to manifest for it to nevertheless be deeply felt. Heavy, stifling atmospheres, environments where you don't feel comfortable, make huge demands on the energy of the lungs. Suffering or sickness in the pulmonary system (nose, throat, bronchia) speak to us then about situations or people who make us ill at ease even though they don't aggress us directly. Something often said by people consulting me is: "I feel like I'm suffocating with that person," or, "I can't breathe in that family." It was in fact an asthmatic person who made this last remark to me and who quickly came to understand who was "sucking the air out of him" in his family.

Excessive maternal anxiety and heavy family atmospheres often turn into pulmonary weaknesses in children. If the child is medicated (suppression of symptoms) the condition can develop into **respiratory or skin allergies**. The child then tries to defend herself by reacting, sometimes violently. **Asthma, eczema,** and **strep throat** are the kinds of cries for attention that express what is taking place in the child: she is experiencing a situation as an aggression, and she needs protection (company and love), but doesn't need to be smothered.

The final meaning associated with pulmonary problems is that of sadness, melancholy, sorrow, and solitude. The energy of the lungs governs these feelings, and if they are excessive they will exhaust this energy. An excess of sadness or the fact that you are cultivating sadness to maintain the memory of something or someone can manifest as chronic weakness in the lungs. Notable examples of this kind of emotional connection come from the Romantic era, the time of Wordsworth, Keats, Byron, Shelley, Chopin, and others, which, not surprisingly, was an era when tuberculosis was rampant.

▸ THE SKIN

This is one of the most fascinating and complete organs of the human body. In fact, it is the only organ directly related to *all* the functions of the body and the mind. This envelope of more than two square yards covers the surface of the body and represents a kind of spread-out brain. It is an extraordinary information system linked directly to the brain that is irrigated and innervated in a remarkable way across its entire surface.

The first role of the skin is that of protection: it protects us from microbial and material aggression (heat, dirt, blows, etc.). It also represents the barrier between us and the external world. You might wonder why I mention the skin in connection with the pulmonary system; it's because the skin supports the cutaneous breathing that assists the lungs in their role of assimilating energy from the air. However, it goes further than a straightforward gaseous exchange because it receives and transforms solar radiation with its action of metabolizing vitamin D. Thanks to more than 700,000 nerve receptors, the skin allows us to feel the environment physically (in the form of touch and temperature) as well as in terms of the human environment (in the form of skin reactions and emotional reactions). The skin also carries out the significant mission of assisting in the body's elimination process. When the kidneys, the urinary bladder, the large intestine, and the lungs are fatigued or overloaded, it is the skin that picks up the slack and helps to clear (notably through perspiration as well as through various dermatoses) toxins that the organism cannot otherwise find ways of eliminating.

The skin and the "skin" of the muscles, the fascia, remember our experiences and our emotions. This allows us to understand why touch and certain techniques of massage and the Taoist techniques of moving energy have astonishing results, in particular with all manifestations of a psychosomatic order.

The skin is the organ of the body that is most representative of the ability to heal. This miracle, the underlying cause of which is unexplained, allows an organism to repair itself, to reconstruct itself in a way that is astonishing both in its strength and its effectiveness. This repair takes place by means of the same process that is connected to the formation and clearing of cancer cells (which explains why cancer can sometimes appear in a recently traumatized area when the healing of physical trauma has occurred in a difficult psychological context).

The social role of the skin is also something that is fundamental. It participates directly in the type and mode of relationship that we have with the world. The more societies and cultures become "disinfected" and the more they distance themselves from life in favor of the intellect and appearances, the more touch becomes something forbidden. I find it amusing that nowadays we can, without compunction, interrupt someone who is speaking, but if we touch or brush up against him or her to take something from the table, we excuse ourself, as if this chance contact was more incongruous and incorrect than the fact of having interrupted the person.

Issues with the Skin

Skin problems are a sign of difficulties experienced in relation to the outside world. **Eczema, psoriasis, dry patches, vitiligo, pimples**—all are manifestations of our reaction to the aggression, real or not, that we feel from the outside world. These disorders allow us to justify or explain away our difficulties with the world, while at the same time allowing us to clear the tension we feel. These issues are all the more meaningful in that they always are located in areas that speak volumes.

Several examples come to mind, the first of them personal. A few months ago I took a trip to the country to visit my parents. I was driving on a road that I knew very well. As I approached a more populated area I became annoyed by a driver who entered traffic by cutting in front of me. Forced to brake hard and of course annoyed about the driver's bad behavior, I flashed my headlights at him. Of course that had the effect of making him angry, and he decided it would be a good idea to slow down to show me who was boss. Instantly regretting my reaction, which was useless anyway, I didn't get into escalating things, but a short distance farther along, having a relatively powerful car, I took advantage of a four-lane section to quickly overtake this driver. However, he too speeded up to prevent me from passing. Since my car was more powerful, I managed nevertheless to pass him, but by accelerating to a speed way beyond what I had intended. Just as I passed him at the end of the four-lane stretch there was a radar trap. I was stopped and ticketed for speeding. It is clear that my feelings of aggression from the external world were very strong that day. The next day, a patch of dry skin appeared on my chest, on my sternum between the solar plexus (raw emotions, aggression, fear) and the cardiac plexus (love of others and oneself, altruism). So long as I had not made peace inside myself over this incident these dry areas were constantly itchy. A homeopathic doctor friend to whom I had confided my story helped me get rid of the rash quickly with a homeopathic remedy that unblocked and emptied my intestines, because he perceived I had trouble clearing the event (large intestine), but also in assimilating it (small intestine).

The second example I'm thinking about is even more striking. One of my students in Taoist practice, Christine, had been suffering since May 1988 with psoriasis. Although every year she took treatments in Israel, at the Dead Sea, the issue would return with more strength each time. This woman, delicate and elegant, suffered greatly from this situation, which led her to cover more and more of herself because her body was more and more affected. Psoriasis is a flaking-off of the skin that presents as reddish blotches that most often appear at the elbows and knees. The tension experienced at these sites is associated with a difficulty in bending, in accepting what is happening. As the skin is the first organ of exchange, it seems this skin issue is trying to say that the exchanges we are having with the external world are unsatisfactory. After some energy sessions, including the identification and liberation of hidden emotional memories, Christine saw her psoriasis diminish and then disappear completely, never to return, in May 1990 (well, what a coincidence that just as it had appeared, it disappeared in May once again).

The Urinary System

The urinary system allows us to manage organic liquids and eliminate toxins from the body. It is made up of the kidneys and the urinary bladder. This is the system that filters, stores, and eliminates "waste water" from our organism, whereas the large intestine eliminates organic matter; so one eliminates solids and the other liquids. This role is fundamental because the body's water is an essential carrier of a person's deep memories. The element of Water, as noted earlier, is intimately linked to ancestral memories. Here we are in the presence of the most profound and powerful activity of the human body—that of the management of "underground water" and of fertility (fecundity).

Issues in the Urinary System

Such issues mean that we are experiencing tension in our deep beliefs, those on which we have constructed our life and that represent our foundation. Problems anywhere in the urinary system mean that we have fear and resistance as we face possible life changes and that we are afraid of being thrown off balance by having to change. Such issues also speak to us of our deepest, most basic fears, such as the fear of death, serious illness, or violence.

▸ THE KIDNEYS

The kidneys are two organs that are essential to the management and filtration of organic liquids and salts in the body. Filtering more than 1,500 liters of blood a day, they sort out and extract toxins from the blood and transform them into urine, which in turn is cleared from the body by means of the urinary bladder. The kidneys regulate the level of water and mineral salts by extracting them from the blood and putting them back based on what is needed. This is how they facilitate the capacity to recover after making physical effort. We will see how this is completely in line with their energetic role as well.

The kidneys play a significant role managing stress and fear. With the participation of the adrenal glands (cortex and medulla), they secrete hormones that determine our behavior in the face of stress and fear. The adrenal medulla secretes adrenaline and noradrenaline, which invokes the fight-or-flight response. The adrenal cortex secretes natural corticosteroids that control the inflammatory level, that is, the level of emotion and passion at the cellular level.

Issues with the Kidneys

The kidneys speak to us about our fears, whether deep and essential (life, death, survival) or related to change. Kidney problems can mean that we are having difficulty letting go of habits or old patterns of thought and belief. Such resistance to change can be due either to fear, insecurity, or a refusal to budge—our stubbornness in refusing to abandon an idea or belief even though everything seems to be leading us in that direction or perhaps even forcing us there. These old, crystallized patterns can manifest as **kidney stones,** a crystallization in the kidneys. Kidney issues are often accompanied by tension or pain in the low back.

Kidney pain can also indicate that we have experienced a situation involving violent and visceral fear (a serious accident, an attack, etc.), in which we are aware of having had a brush with death or have seen death up close. In such instances the hair, which depends energetically on the kidneys, can suddenly turn white.

Finally, kidney problems can express our difficulty finding stability in life, finding the proper balance of activity, aggression, and defense, which belong to the left kidney, and passivity, listening, and flight, which belong to the right kidney. This is why kidney issues sometimes let us know about our difficulty deciding things in life, and then our difficulty in doing what is needed so that what we have decided actually happens.

▸ **THE URINARY BLADDER**

The urinary bladder receives, stores, and eliminates organic liquids loaded with toxins that are entrusted to it by the kidneys. This management of urine is far from being as trifling as it might appear because if the bladder does not play its role, the body will completely poison itself. The bladder is to the urinary system what the large intestine is to the digestive system. It is the last stage in the process of the management and elimination of organic liquids and, by extension, the energetic clearing of old memories.

Urinary Bladder Issues

Such issues are a sign of difficulty in clearing our "waste water," that is, old memories that are no longer satisfying. Old beliefs, old habits, patterns of thought unsuited to the present situation are the kind of memories that poison the mind just as toxins do the body. When the energies of the bladder are functioning as they should, these emotional toxins are eliminated with no problem. In contrast, tension and pain tell us that things aren't going so well. It means that we're afraid of letting go or changing our habits, beliefs, patterns, or ways of thinking and acting. Too great an attachment to memories, whether they are satisfactory or not, sometimes leads us to be stuck in life. These situations show up as various forms of tension in the bladder. **UTIs** (urinary tract infections) or other inflammations speak to us about this, telling us that we are holding anger or some other deep-seated emotion connected to memories.

Bladder trouble can also mean that we have difficulties overcoming deep-seated fears in relation to our ancestors. Young boys who are afraid of their parents (justified or not), and especially fear of the father (or a father figure or father substitute such as a grandparent or teacher) often express it in **bedwetting** (enuresis). Girls tend to express the same fears in repeated UTIs.

The Circulatory System

This system is in charge of the circulation of blood throughout the body. Thanks to this system the precious liquid that is our blood is able to circulate and nourish with oxygen and nutrients even the tiniest and most remote part of our organism. And it is this circulation that permits the blood to play its role of purification because it transports toxins rejected by the cells and eliminates carbon dioxide being exchanged with oxygen. The circulatory function then is about distributing blood, which represents life, to all parts of the body, and by extension bringing the joy of life. The circulatory system is made up of the heart, the venous system, and the arterial system. It runs through the organism by describing a kind of figure eight, as seen in chapter 1, figure 1.1, which represents the Earlier Heaven and Later Heaven, the conscious and the nonconscious—what a coincidence!

Issues in the Circulatory System

Circulatory problems mean that we are having trouble letting life circulate freely in ourself, and that our joy in life, our love of life, is having trouble being expressed or even existing in/inside us. What part of ourself have we been neglecting to love to such an extent that we are not even letting life itself—in the form of blood—nourish it? What part of life are we rejecting? What emotional trauma has entered so that we no longer have any room for joy or love? Why are we afraid? These are questions that our inner master can send us through tension and problems in the circulatory system.

▸ THE HEART

The heart is the principal blood circulation organ. It is the master pump for the circulation, and moreover an intelligent and autonomous pump with an extraordinary sensitivity in its responses. Through its rhythm it is capable of responding instantaneously to the slightest demand, whether it is physiological (effort) or psychological (emotion). In close relationship with the brain it is capable of very precise regulation of the circulatory pressure and rhythm required by environmental circumstances. The heart is what orders and directs our ability to adapt inner reactions to external necessities. The heart muscle is involuntary, meaning it operates outside our conscious will. Its relationship with our nonconscious is strong, and this explains the important influence conscious and unconscious emotions have on cardiac rhythm. Traditionally considered the seat of love and the emotions, its privileged relationship with the brain, which depends on the heart energetically, shows us how much true love cannot be limited to being passionate but must also be intelligent, otherwise it risks being blind.

Issues in the Heart

Heart-related issues speak to us about difficulties experiencing love and managing our emotions, which have a tendency to take over life. They can also mean that we are giving too much space to resentment, hatred, and violence, which we are either repressing or expressing indirectly (through sports, games, and so forth). During such times the space available for love of life, love of ourself, love of others, or love of what we are doing diminishes day by day. Remember that the heart distributes blood inside us. If we cultivate negative emotional states, they are going to get distributed in the same way. In energy work we say that the state of the heart and its Shen (its spiritual representation) shows in the complexion of the person and in the brilliance of her eyes, in her gaze.

Palpitations, tachycardia, heart attack, and other cardiac problems express all the troubles we have in managing emotional states, or if we've repressed our emotions, in letting them be expressed or have a life within us. Taking life and everything that happens too seriously, the lack of pleasure in what we do or feel, the lack of space for free time and relaxation—all these conditions weaken the energies of the heart and can convert into cardiac tension. However, an excess of pleasure or passion can also weaken the energies of the heart and can result in the same kinds of effects.

▶ THE VENOUS SYSTEM

This is the system usually represented as blue in the anatomy charts many of us have seen at one time or another. The venous system carries worn-out blood to the liver and kidneys for it to be filtered, and carries blood to the lungs to clear carbon dioxide and have it recharged with oxygen. This is the yin part of the circulatory system, the part that receives and preserves. Through its alveoli and its ability to dilate, the venous system has a passive, yin action within the circulation.

Issues in the Venous System

Venous system problems express a difficulty in accepting or receiving life, the joy of living, or love, and our difficulty in leaving room for these things in ourself. We are having trouble with stagnating emotions. The experience is felt as a kind of dullness, a lack of passion, and a joylessness. There is a sensation of not knowing how or feeling incapable of making our desire for happiness come alive in ourself and in our relationships with others. Consequently, the emotions stagnate in us, creating a feeling of despondency and powerlessness. **Phlebitis** and **varicose veins** express our feelings of being obliged to accept things that prevent us from being really happy.

▶ THE ARTERIAL SYSTEM

In those same anatomy charts most of us have seen, this is the system that appears in red. The arterial system transports blood enriched with oxygen and nutrients to the organs and cells. This is the yang part of our circulatory system that engages active assistance from the heart in the circulation. Through its ability to contract and expand, called *vaso-constriction* and *vasodilation,* the arterial system, in fact, helps the work of the heart.

Issues in the Arterial System

Such issues speak to us about tensions that are equivalent to those that appear in the venous system, but in the active sense. The emotions involved are excessive and manifest in excess (joviality, excitement, etc.), or else they are held back, stifled. The difficulty or more likely the inability to do what is needed in life in order to feel joy, pleasure, or happiness gets converted into **high blood pressure** (hypertension). In contrast to problems in the venous system, where we feel we are prevented from experiencing happiness, problems in the arterial system indicate we don't know how, aren't able, or have been unable to make room for love and the joy of living.

High blood pressure reveals tension due to an excessive will to search for the experience of love and happiness, but fear prevents this, which causes internal pressure. Everything takes on excessive proportions and that frightens us. The fear crystallizes in us and hardens the walls of the arteries, thereby increasing, through **arterioscle-rosis,** the phenomenon of tension. One of the deep fears associated with hypertension is the fear of death. We're afraid that death will arrive before we've done all we have to do. A feeling of urgency then develops and "pushes the pressure" even higher. Here too we find connections with homeopathy, which uses the remedy ACONITE to treat hypertension as well as the fear of death and all things that are based on panic.

Low blood pressure (hypotension), on the other hand, speaks to us of defeat, of feeling like a victim. Conquered by events with no way out, we are no longer able to push the pressure up to get the machine going again. The underlying dynamic is passive, and discouragement prevails over the sense of struggle. No doubt we have missed out on love in our life, the food that facilitates joy and a reason for living, for feeling our heart beating. This flame is missing or perhaps we have not maintained it.

The Nervous System

The nervous system can be considered our body's tertiary system. It is the control and management center for information. It centralizes, stores, restores, and circulates data that is innate or acquired by the person, allowing him to exist and evolve in his environment. It is clear for each one of us that the role of the nervous system is essential and that it participates in even the tiniest of our organism's activities. It is divided into two parts: the central nervous system and the autonomic nervous system. Organically it is made up of the brain, the marrow of the spine, and the nerves (peripheral, sympathetic, and parasympathetic).

▸ THE CENTRAL NERVOUS SYSTEM

This system manages thought, conscious movement, and all sensation. It is made up of the brain, the spinal marrow, and the peripheral nerves. All conscious thought, all decisions, and all voluntary actions pass through the central nervous system.

Issues with the Central Nervous System

Nervous-system issues are a sign of difficulty in consciously and intellectually managing our life and our emotions. Harshness, too much work, a tendency to experience and resolve things through thinking and not through feeling will manifest as unbalance, illness, or tension in the central nervous system. More severely, **epilepsy,** with its moments of brief unconscious behavior, termed *automatism,* represents a disconnection of the central nervous system in favor of the autonomic nervous system.

▸ THE BRAIN

The brain is the central computer of the body. This is where thoughts are developed, where most information is stored, and where conscious decisions are made. The brain is divided in several ways. The first way is the division into two hemispheres, the right hemisphere and the left hemisphere. The left is in charge of thought, reasoning, logic, and language. It manages everything having to do with the rational, the conscious, and the intentional. It principally controls everything on the right side of the body (hand, leg, etc.). The right hemisphere is in charge of the imagination, artistic sense and creativity, spatial awareness, intuition, affects, and memory, whether it is auditory, visual, or sensory. It manages everything having to do with the irrational, the unconscious, and the involuntary. It principally controls everything on the left side of the body (hand, leg, etc.). I would like to make quite clear, however, that this inverse control involves only the motor activities of the body and not the manifestation of symptoms, as this is a very common cause for errors of interpretation.

The second way of dividing up the brain refers to the "three brains," an idea that derives from the work of French surgeon and philosopher Henri Laborit (1914–1995). There is the so-called reptilian brain, the brain of instinct, reflex actions, as well as life rhythms and survival. This is the first brain, the oldest in our understanding of evolution. Next is the so-called limbic brain, the brain of emotions, adaptation to the surrounding environment, relationships with others, and the filtering of perceived information. Finally, there is the cerebral cortex or neocortex, the brain of reflection, analysis, abstraction, creation, and imagination. Through this three-brained structure we can see human evolution in three phases: animal, emotive and social, and finally analytical and creative.

Finally, the third way of dividing up the brain refers to "five brains," a concept proposed by American creativity researcher and author Ned Hermann (1922–1999). Hermann took into account the first two ways of dividing up the brain and integrated them. We can compare this to the sacral vertebrae, which are 3 + 2, and the lumbar vertebrae, which are 5. We have the reptilian brain, the brain of instinct; the right limbic brain, which is in charge of emotionality and spirituality; the left limbic brain, which is in charge of organization and down-to-earthness; the right neocortex, which manages synthesis and creativity; and finally the left neocortex, which manages logic and technique. Notably we find a direct relationship between these five brains and the Five Principles of Chinese medicine. The reptilian brain corresponds to the element Metal, the right limbic brain to Fire, the left limbic brain to Water, the right neocortex to Wood, and the left neocortex to Earth.

That said, it is essential to understand that these ways of dividing up the brain are analytical and explanatory. They identify the main characteristics of the brain, but they do not in any way correspond to the way the brain is divided up physically or functionally. All functions and parts of the brain are closely related to one another, are in continuous interaction, and participate in the same cerebral dynamic.

Issues in the Brain

Cerebral problems are a sign of difficulty in managing situations in life that require us to use our thinking. The "conscious consciousness" dominates and tries to regulate or understand everything, but it doesn't succeed. Our relationship to life is built on reason, rational logic, and reasoning. Tension or pathology in the brain expresses the intention of setting things straight using thought, coolly and without emotion. We don't get emotional or we don't get tangled up in possible emotions that might be parasitical either because we're afraid of them or because they don't satisfy us and they seem useless. Only direct and visible effectiveness counts, often understood and materialized by the management and financial side of life.

Thinking about everything in terms of profitability at the expense of the human side, so characteristic of the present-day business environment, often shows up in people as cerebral problems starting with simple **migraines** and going up the scale to **vertigo,** troubles with **concentration and memory, circulatory problems,** and ending up sometimes with **tumors, heart attack,** or **stroke.** *Karoshi* is a Japanese term that refers to death by overworking. This total disjuncture due to overwork, commonly called "burnout" in the West, is currently ravaging Japan, killing thousands of people, and is now beginning to appear in Europe as well. The term *burnout* is notable when we connect it to the fact that we are talking about the Fire principle. These manifestations of imbalance in our connection to life appear most often in white-collar or intellectual professions, and are much rarer in people who have manual or physical professions that oblige them to remain connected with real life, expressions of the Earth principle.

Imbalances in the brain speak to us about difficulties making room for pleasure and simple joy in life. This underscores the relationship between the brain and the heart, which manages the brain at an energetic level. When rational thinking dominates, it implies the need to be right all the time and making mistakes is a sign of weakness. But this means that we are rejecting the human component of error—its necessity and its experimental and evolutionary dimension—retaining from it only the concept of fault and therefore, guilt. This kind of imbalance can manifest as tension in the brain, migraines, and headaches.

▸ THE SPINAL MARROW

The spinal marrow is the part of the nervous system that descends within the spinal column. It transmits cervical data and instructions to all parts of the body. It has some autonomy in that certain reflexes (the reflex in the knees, for example) are controlled directly by it. The spinal marrow, constructed of both nerve fiber (white matter) and neurons (gray matter), makes use of a looping system. This loop system means that a pain stimulus, for example, does not have to go all the way to the brain to provoke a muscular reaction; the information coming from the affected area goes directly to the muscle concerned.

Issues with the Spinal Marrow

Such issues show us how we are prevented from transforming our ideas and thoughts into reality. Problems here express our difficulty in acting or even reacting, that is, without thinking about it in relation to a given context. Finally, spinal marrow issues speak to us about our refusal to let life and the joy of being alive express themselves through our acts or our reactions. **Paralysis, myelitis,** and **cerebrospinal meningitis** prevent us from acting or reacting, from doing—therefore preventing us from being mistaken or making mistakes.

▶ THE NERVES

The nerves are our personal "cabling system" that allow our central computer, the brain, to be connected to our peripherals, the organs, muscles, five senses, and so forth. In the central nervous system the nerves are of two types, sensitive and motor. The sensitive nerves transmit perceived information to the brain or the spinal marrow. The motor nerves transmit orders from the brain or the spinal marrow to the affected part of the body

Issues with the Nerves

Nerve problems express difficulty in moving thoughts, desires, or wishes into reality. The transmission gives out and orders no longer work. "What is it that I don't want to do?" or "What am I afraid of doing?" or "What is paralyzing me?" These are the kinds of questions expressed by pain or blockages in the nervous system. A typical case is that of **paralyzing sciatica,** in which the sciatic nerve is completely blocked and prevents the person from walking, moving around, or even just standing (refer to the section on the lower limbs in chapter 4). Depending on the side affected, what is happening in our relational life? Who is it that we no longer want to move toward, with whom do we no longer want to have the kind of relationship we have at present, or no relationship at all?

Cruralgia is notable in this regard because its pinching of the crural nerve manifests among other ways in men, through sometimes very debilitating pain in one of the two testicles. In women, the pain will manifest in the ovaries. The same issues I mentioned above for paralyzing sciatica can provide especially informative responses, even though they may not be necessarily welcome or accepted. In any case we can see how the location of the affected nerve informs us precisely about the deeper, underlying nature of the condition. We need only take a look at the part of the body concerned to be able to make a connection between the two.

▸ THE AUTONOMIC NERVOUS SYSTEM

Also called the neurovegetative system, this system is in charge of all of a person's unconscious activity. Organic functions (e.g., blood circulation, digestion, breathing), but also psychological, emotional, or defense functions (e.g., goosebumps, vomiting, blushing, flight-or-fight response), depend on this system. Whereas the central nervous system is connected to striated muscle tissue, the autonomic system is connected to smooth muscle tissue. The autonomic system includes the parasympathetic system and the sympathetic system. The parasympathetic system is in charge of all those things having to do with routines in the organism such as organic functions, whereas the sympathetic system is in charge of activities of excitement and defense and emergency, such as the fight-or-flight response. The autonomic system is managed by the hypothalamus and the medulla oblongata.

Issues in the Autonomic Nervous System

Imbalances in this system express difficulties in connecting the conscious and the nonconscious. These issues tell us that our nonconscious is having trouble managing requests coming from the external world, notably emotions. What happens then is a phenomenon of saturation of the central nervous system that is no longer able to direct our physical activity because the autonomic system has taken over. The autonomic system requires us to make or not make a certain number of moves or actions or else it prevents us from accessing certain levels of consciousness or memory. All the manifestations of **hyperventilation syndrome,** such as **trembling, nervous tics, nausea, migraines, cramps,** and **tetany** are expressions of this difficulty of controlling and responding correctly to requests from the external world.

The Reproductive System

As its name indicates this system allows the human being to reproduce. It is made up of the sexual organs, sexual glands (testicles, ovaries), and in women the uterus. In this highly developed system the human lineage is perpetuated through the penetration by a man, the yang principle, of a woman, the yin principle. The nature of yang is to penetrate; the nature of yin is to be receptive. Thus life shows us to what extent evolution is only possible through the meeting of opposites. By observing life we can begin to understand how important it is to unite the yin and yang principles within ourself to foster our own evolution. We need to move forward and encounter the other aspect of ourself—the feminine/yin aspect if we are men, and the yang/masculine aspect if we are women. We're not speaking about sexuality here of course, but instead about what C. G. Jung calls the *anima* (feminine) and the *animus* (masculine). This is about the feminine side that is gentle, tender, passive, artistic, aesthetic, welcoming, unconscious, and deep, and about the masculine side that is firm, strong, active, defensive, penetrating, conscious, and superficial. It is possible for us to grow, evolve, and gradually attain what I call "the peace of opposites" (which Jung termed the "reconciliation of opposites"), thereby arriving at union within.

What is noteworthy is that it is completely possible for this (pro) creation to take place in pleasure and joy (orgasmic enjoyment), just as life has provided for us. This should be pondered by those whose course of personal development unfolds in intention and strength, or in constraint and urgency.

The reproductive system allows us to procreate, to give new life physically. By extension this also has to do with our general ability to create or give birth in the material world (to projects, ideas, etc.). It is also the system of sexuality, the ability to create in climactic enjoyment. It represents our action on others, on the person with whom we are engaged, and our power over that person because that person abandons himself to us as we do to him in this specific relationship. This power needs to be reciprocal and respectful, and it is much greater when it is supported by love. With love and respect, this exercise of power over each other can be positive and a source of great pleasure in life, as it is normally punctuated by orgasm. Orgasm represents the supreme climactic enjoyment of creation, of the creative and procreative act shared with another person. When love and respect are lacking, however, the exercise of sexual power can lead to competition, power struggles, or a resigned attitude that causes a person to engage in sexual union out of a sense of duty.

Issues in the Reproductive System

Such issues speak to us of difficulties experiencing or accepting this "peace of opposites" within ourself. The issues can manifest in various ways, but they always mean that there is tension with another person, either a spouse or a child or their representatives within us or outside of us. This is especially the case when there are problems in the uterus, which represents the home and the nest, and often means tension or suffering in relation to the spouse (e.g., absence, frustration, death, conflict) or in relation to the position of each person within the home.

These issues also express our fear—the fear of producing a child, whether it is an actual child or a symbolic one in the form of a project, idea, and so forth. The fear can be anchored in a lack of confidence, guilt, or anxiety. Pain in the testicles or ovaries speaks to us about this, in the appearance of **cruralgia, cysts,** or **cancer** in these reproductive areas. **Sexually transmitted diseases (STDs)** often represent self-punishment unconsciously provoked though guilt when confronting sexual activity that is elaborated outside the norms recognized by the person or his or her culture or religion. This guilt, conscious or not, leads the person to punish himself or herself through what I might boldly call a "slipup," in which the person sexually encounters a man or woman who is going to transmit to her or him a "shameful disease."

In the case of **frigidity, impotency,** or pain and various inflammations that prevent sexual activity we are expressing a difficulty in experiencing the pleasures of life, in particular the pleasures of activity, whether that activity is professional, social, or within the family. We don't allow ourself to experience enjoyment, satisfaction, or even climactic pleasure as we exercise our personal power over things or over others. All of that seems too serious or guilt-inducing and we no longer know how to experience the simple, childlike joy of having done something that works and that we're proud of. We believe that this power is shameful or negative when it can be creative and fertile because what gives it the positive or negative coloring is the use that we make of it and the intention that we put into it, in the same way that the power we give to love and sexuality can create or destroy, liberate or alienate, animate or close down the other person and ourself.

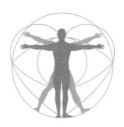

6

The Sense Organs and Other Conditions of the Body

Feedback from the Inner Master

A man who doesn't know how to cry, is not a man.

ARCHIE FIRE LAME DEER

In the previous chapters we discussed the main parts of the body and how they speak to us, as well as the major systems of the body. We will now look at all the components of the head and face, as well as at some specific conditions by which our inner master communicates to us.

The Head and Face: Symbol of Identity and Seat of the Sense Organs

The head and face assemble the five senses—sight, hearing, smell, taste, and touch. While representing our identity, the face is also the honored seat of "fine" perception of the external world—the perception of color, sound, taste, odor, and temperature. We perceive these sensations through our refined material world sensors—the eyes, ears, nose, mouth, and skin. These sense organs make it possible for us to perceive complex levels of the material world. However, through any problems that arise in the sense organs, we also express the energetic blockages or resistance we might have toward recognizing or accepting what we perceive.

General, problems of the face speak to us about problems of identity, about difficulties accepting our identity. Conditions such as **acne, eczema,** and **red patches** fall into this category, but so do certain facial characteristics such as a **beard** or **mustache** express the ways we demonstrate difficulties in accepting our face, either because we don't like it or because it is attractive and generates more attention than we want to receive. There are various ways of hiding the face or making it ugly so that it changes or rejects an identity image that we're not pleased with.

▶ THE EYES AND RELATED ISSUES

The eyes are the organs of vision. With the eyes we see the world in color (the representation of feeling) and with depth perception (the representation of structure). This ability depends on our having two eyes. The right eye, which represents the person's structure and is yin, provides "horizontal" vision. The left eye, which represents the personality and is yang, provides "vertical" vision. Both eyes together give us global vision. The eyes are associated with the energy of the element Wood; therefore they represent the level of perception that is most related to feelings and to *being*. This helps us understand why many cases of **nearsightedness** appear in adolescence, (as well as **scoliosis,** described in chapter 4), as this is the period of life when a child begins to extend her affective bearings in relation to the external world, beyond the family structure.

Issues with the eyes therefore mean that we're having difficulty seeing something in our life, specifically, something that touches us emotionally. "What don't I want to see?" "What brings into question my very being or brings into question the position that I accord it?" Frequently this kind of questioning is associated with a deep feeling of injustice. If we're dealing with the right eye, the tension is related to yin, maternal symbolism, and if it's the left eye what we are refusing to see is related to yang, paternal symbolism.

Let's return to the case of Pascal that I brought up in the previous chapter in connection with the femur issues (see page 111). To review, at the age of nine and a half, he lost his father to a car accident that occurred while his father was working. This disappearance of the male pillar in Pascal's life had to be accepted as a fact by his conscious mind and in his thinking, but he could not accept it on the level of the nonconscious. On his next birthday, at the age of ten, six months after the disappearance, the child's left eye began to swell up aggressively. Even with hospitalization and multiple tests, the medical staff could find nothing wrong with the boy. The doctors, speaking in front of the child, who wasn't expected to understand, decided to operate the next day "to see what was going on with the eye." The next morning, upon awakening, it was discovered that the edema had completely disappeared. Clearly, the child had refused to "see," (to perceive something in relation to the yang [father]) that is, to accept his father's death. His fear about the pending surgical intervention caused him to immediately halt the expression of the tension between his conscious and his nonconscious. Instead, the boy stifled the emotion. However, several years later, at the age of twenty-eight, he had his own car accident as he was coming home from work (just like his father), in which he fractured his left femur. The accident occurred during a period in which Pascal was experiencing a difficult phase of conflict and flight in relation to anything representing forms of authority, whether social or familial. He was reliving, without being aware of it, what he had experienced at the time of his father's death, that is, "What is my place, who am I, nobody understands me or helps me, why this injustice?"

Each type of ocular manifestation conveys a specific message:

Myopia (nearsightedness), the difficulty in seeing at a distance, represents the unconscious fear of the future, which looks blurry (i.e., not well defined or fuzzy).

Cataracts, which are characterized by a clouding or even a complete loss of vision, express a fear of the present or the future, which appears dark.

Presbyopia (farsightedness), difficulty seeing objects that are close, represents a fear of seeing what is present or in the near future. This condition mainly affects older people and is parallel to age-related memory loss, which follows the same process in terms of remembering recent events less and less, and more distant events more and more. Farsightedness is associated notably with the approach of death, which represents an end date that we might not want to see.

Astigmatism is the condition of not seeing objects exactly as they are, but rather in a distorted and blurry way. This condition symbolizes a difficulty in seeing things as they are.

▶ THE EARS AND RELATED ISSUES

Ears are the organs of hearing. They allow us to capture, receive, and then transmit sound messages in encoded form. Ears are connected to the Water element and, by extension, to our origins. Auriculotherapists can "read" in the ear the form of an inverted fetus, and according to Chinese wisdom it is possible to see if a person is an old soul, one who has had many incarnated lifetimes.* The Creator's sound (described in Genesis with the sentence, "In the beginning was the Word") was the first manifestation of form. Our ears connect us to our divine origins. Tibetan Buddhists say that the last sense to go upon death is that of sound. The ears are the representation of our capacity for listening, integrating, and accepting what comes to us from outside sources.

Ear problems, including **buzzing, tinnitus,** and partial, selective, or total **deafness** are signs that we are having trouble hearing (or even

---

*Auriculotherapy, or ear acupuncture, is based on the premise that the ears are a microcosm of the entire body, such that conditions affecting the physical, mental, or emotional health of a person are treated by stimulation of the surface of the ear.

that we refuse to hear) what is going on around us. If the deafness is on the right side it is connected to maternal/yin symbolism, and if on the left, with paternal/yang symbolism. For example, this was the case with Raphael, who kept having ear infections in his right ear. Not surprisingly, his mother had a tendency to shout a lot, and the child couldn't stand the constant yelling.

▶ THE MOUTH AND RELATED ISSUES

The mouth allows us to both nourish and express ourself. It is an open doorway between the inner and outer worlds through which we receive food and, by extension, life experiences, which are psychological food. This doorway works in the other direction as well, from the inside to the outside, being the orifice by which we express (including spitting or vomiting) what is inside and needs to leave.

The mouth belongs to the Earth element and to the digestive system (the yin phase); it also expresses the Metal element in its role in the respiratory system (the yang phase). It is the doorway through which Earth energies (in the form of food and experiences) and the energies of Heaven (air, breath, understanding) penetrate us to become our essential energy (as described in chapter 2). The mouth's connection to the Earth element and to the digestive system indicates its vital role in nutrition, both physical nutrition, as food, and psychological nutrition, as experiences. Teeth symbolize the ability to more easily "bite" into life and "chew" what life offers, to be swallowed and digested. Newborn babies and the elderly cannot do this; the only foods they are capable of swallowing must be liquid or near liquid, or, from the psychological perspective, emotional.

Problems in the mouth are a sign of difficulties in "biting" into life, in accepting what life offers and in "chewing" it to improve our assimilation of it. **Cold sores, inflammation in the mouth, cheek or tongue bites** are all signs that what is being offered to us or what we are being told does not satisfy us. Problems in this area can also mean that the education that we are given and the experiences that we encounter are not to our taste, that we're not pleased about them. They represent difficulties in accepting new tastes, that is, new ideas, opinions, and experiences. However, they can also be a sign of saturation, of too much experience, and by extension, of the need to take a break.

▸ THE NOSE AND RELATED ISSUES

The nose is the orifice through which air penetrates the body and by which we perceive odors, that is, what emanates from the manifest world. The nose and the sense of smell belong to the Metal element. We breathe through the nose; through it we allow the energy of the air in the form of the breath (Heaven) to enter us. The level of assimilation of energies through the nose is therefore finer than the level in the mouth, which is concerned with the assimilation of a coarser level of matter. And yet the mouth is closely connected to the nose through the sense of smell, which is an essential partner of taste. The connection of smell to taste is as important as the connection between the two eyes.

Issues related to the nose speak to us about the fear of allowing the finer dimensions of life in. This specifically concerns intimacy and the acceptance of intimate information about ourself or others. For example, odor plays an important role in sexuality, whether it be vegetable, animal, or human sexuality. **Sinusitis, stuffy nose,** or **loss of the sense of smell** are typical signs of difficulties in accepting intimate information that makes its way to us. It displeases us because it "smells bad." What smells bad? Well, poop and pus do, not flowers. "What is the 'poop' of my life?" "What stinks in my life?" These are the kind of questions we must ask ourself. Each time we say to someone, "I can't feel it" or "I can't see it," think of the mirror effect and reflect on what part of oneself is being brought back to us by what we are unwilling to sense or see. Issues with odors no doubt express rancor, bitterness, or a desire for revenge that we are letting rot in us. Nose issues can mean that our fear of life's manifestations and particularly our animal nature is great, since life is also excrement, death, and decay. We can't tolerate these last three because we place value judgments on them. Perhaps we too easily forget that the nicest vegetables and the most beautiful flowers grow on manure or compost, and that life finds its nourishment from death, which is not an end to life, but a transition to another form of life.

▶ **THE THROAT AND RELATED ISSUES**

The throat is the portal through which we ingest both nourishment and air. Two feeding conduits comprise the throat: the esophagus (material food) and the trachea (air). The throat is also where the vocal chords and tonsils are located. At the front of the throat in the laryngeal hollow is located a fundamental gland, the thyroid. A very elaborate reflex system allows us to select the type of "food," whether solid or air, and direct it toward the appropriate vessel, either the stomach or the lungs. When the distinguishing mechanism of the throat isn't working properly we choke or swallow air. By means of the vocal cords the throat is the vehicle and medium of oral expression. Speech, words, or cries depend on the throat. Ultimately, the throat is the gatekeeper that filters and selects all the comings and goings of the body. As for the thyroid, we might say that it is the principal gland regulating growth and human metabolism as well as the development of the physical body (growth and weight).

In energy work the throat is considered the seat of the all-important throat chakra, the center of self-expression and one of the ways we position ourself in relation to the external world. The throat chakra represents our ability to recognize and express who and what we are and to receive what can enrich us, nourish us, and make us grow. Finally, it is the seat of our potential for expressing creativity. Issues with the throat are expressions of "What is stuck in my throat?" Throat issues also concern acceptance, as in "What is it that I can't manage to swallow?"

Loss of voice, sore throat, having food go down the wrong way, and **swallowing air** are some of the signs of difficulties expressing what we think or feel, often out of a fear of the consequences, so we prefer instead to self-censor. Throat issues are also signs of a lack of self-expression, expression of who and what one is, of one's qualities and weaknesses. "What am I not managing to get through, to say?" **Hyperthyroidism,** a yang condition, and **hypothyroidism,** a yin condition, are often signs of an impossibility of saying or doing what one wants to say or do. Nobody can understand us, we don't have the means of getting across what we believe or want to say, we are afraid that the other person will not accept what we would like to say, or we are afraid of the strength or the violence of what might come out of us if we said what we really want to say. Behind all these forms of nonexpression there is always the idea of risk, of danger, which stops us and makes us hold back our expression. The yang form manifests a desire despite everything to try to express, whereas the yin form expresses an abandonment when faced with the impossibility of expression.

Specific Conditions

▶ ALLERGIES

Allergies are excessive defense reactions when an organism is confronted with an external agent, normally something quite ordinary that has no specific risk, but which is perceived as an aggressor, an enemy. Dust, pollen, mites, perfume, certain foods—these are just some of the substances that an organism can have a reaction to in order to destroy them or drive them out.

Hay fever as well as **skin, digestive,** or **respiratory allergies** speak to us about our difficulty in managing the external world, which is perceived as dangerous or aggressive. We are in defense mode; we are being aggressed—but we are also Joan of Arc leading the charge. We are going to hound that aggressor right out of us! Allergies signify that we are reactive as we confront others, and our first reflex, no matter what is happening, is a strong defensive attitude and sometimes even a strongly reactive attitude. We are active and have decided to protect ourself at all costs. This is why allergy sufferers rarely develop cancer.

▶ AUTOIMMUNE CONDITIONS

These are diseases in which the organism tries to mix several processes all at the same time: it tries to maintain allergies, inflammation, and a cancerous dynamic. These are defense-mechanism illnesses in which the organism no longer recognizes its own cells and begins to fight them and destroy them, considering them dangerous foreign agents. For example, rheumatoid arthritis is degenerative in the sense that it no longer respects the natural laws of organic recognition.

Autoimmune conditions speak about an inability to recognize ourself, to see and accept ourself *as we are*. This difficulty in identifying who and what we are is often aggravated by a search for external sources. We struggle against a world that does not understand us, does not recognize us, does not like us—whereas it's really our own way of perceiving that is the problem. We think of life in a Manichean way in that things are either good or bad, or situations are either right or wrong. This is innately a conflict-oriented and compulsive defense mode that leads us to destroy ourself while believing that we are destroying the world in order to defend ourself—all the time thinking that we are not doing any harm. (See the example of Dominique in chapter 4.)

▶ CANCER, CANCEROUS TUMORS

These diseases have to do with the proliferation of anarchic cells that appear and develop in a given part of the organism. If they are detected in time, the disease can be confined to where it began; otherwise metastasis will occur. The organism will then be progressively invaded by the cancerous cells, which travel through the circulatory system and colonize various parts of the body by means of a kind of "burglary" of the surrounding cellular region.

Given the seriousness of this disease I will list the main characteristics of its process:

- "Underground" disorder, unconscious and painless at the beginning

- Anarchic development through a loss of cellular orientation
- Contamination of the organism through the blood and lymph systems
- Invasion of the organism through colonization
- Colonization through "breaking and entering" the affected areas
- Fatal outcome through self-destruction if there is no intervention

Here we have a description of the entire psychological process that precedes cancer and prepares the ground for its physical manifestation. One day the person undergoes a serious emotional/feeling trauma (or an accumulation of feelings), and he tucks it away in the depths of himself. Through force of will, education, or belief, or out of pure avoidance he does not really recognize his suffering or allow it to be expressed, and more importantly he does not allow or recognize the loss of orientation and the deep destruction of beliefs that it represents. The trauma is deeply felt as an intrusion, a "burglary" of his internal structures, and the resulting shock wave will little by little colonize the whole psychological structure of the person. Little by little the person loses all of his reference points, which become chaotic and "suicidal" for the structure of the person (the opposite of the allergic person, who rarely develops cancer). This whole process spreads by contaminating the person's ability to find joy in life. The emotions, represented by the circulatory system, will little by little become impregnated with the memory of the trauma and will progressively give way to feelings that eventually will undermine the body. All this remains unconscious, underground, and painless—that is, up to the day when everything explodes and bursts into the light of day in the form of cancer.

Cancer is then the destruction of our inner programming that keeps things in balance, and it is expressed through the first area that is affected. It often is a transformation of remorse or wounds that one cannot heal or does not want to heal, which are often associated with guilt. It is often a kind of self-punishment that intends to be definitive—an unconscious realization of failure in the face of one's life or one's choices in life. "What did I lose out on?" "What am I punishing myself for?" "What is it that I blame myself so deeply for?" These are the questions one must ask. In any case, we are in the presence of the final cry shouted out by the inner master because all the other previous cries have failed to get a response or were stifled.

▸ CYSTS AND NODULES

These are small formations of organic liquids or flesh imprisoned in the skin or in body tissue. Most of the time benign, these small balls or pockets represent hardenings or solidifications of emotional memories. They speak to us of a tendency to retain, maintain, and harden certain inner wounds. Rancor, being unable to forget or accept the hardships of life, the hardening of memories that we can't let go of, wounds or frustrations that the ego doesn't accept—these are all the kinds of experiences and feelings that can express themselves as cysts or nodules. Insofar as they are emotional memories, things of the ego, they are very often related to social or professional experiences. The location of the cyst or nodule of course gives us additional information about the type of blocked memory.

▸ HAIR

Hair is governed by the Water element. Losing hair or losing its color are linked to a significant experience of stress, an intense fear connected with death, the fragility of life, and the precarious nature of things. Present-day situations of professional insecurity are behind a growing number of cases of hair loss, which not so long ago used to be something only men suffered from, but nowadays women are experiencing the same professional stress and are also losing hair.

▸ HEADACHES AND MIGRAINES

These often represent difficulties in accepting certain thoughts, ideas, or feelings that bother or constrain us. Stress, setbacks, being assailed by or preyed on by "undesirable" ideas or exterior constraints are the kinds of tension that manifest in the form of headaches and migraine.

When a headache follows a path on each side of the head starting at the nape of neck and ending near the temples or the sides of the eyes, or even directly in an eye, it is called a *hepatobiliary migraine*. Here the tension is of an emotional nature or the experience of a situation is emotional. These kinds of headaches relate to family or intimate partners. When the headache is in the forehead it expresses a rejection of thoughts, a stubbornness about ideas that are present and active. These headaches are related to the professional or social world and the demands this world puts on us.

▸ HYPERVENTILATION
See the entry on the autonomic nervous system on page 161 in the previous chapter.

▸ INFLAMMATION AND FEVER
We have Fire in us and it burns and purifies, producing a heat that destroys. **Tendinitis, fever,** and **inflammation** are there to tell us that we have Fire in us, that there is overheating and excessive or inappropriate use of the part of the body concerned. However, as with allergies, the organism is active, and through the Fire that it is releasing it seeks to alert, to clean, to purify the affected area. The meaning of inflammation must always be connected to the body location where it occurs.

For example, Laurie came to see me about a tendinitis of the right elbow. This inflammation was expressing a difficulty in accepting the fact that her daughter had grown up and was no longer behaving the way she, her mother, wanted. However, she kept insisting and unconsciously pressuring her daughter, who "understood nothing," her mother said, and continued to live her life the way she wanted to. Once Laurie could accept the situation her tendinitis disappeared.

▸ LOW-BACK PAIN (LUMBAGO)
Lumbago is pain or tension in the lower back in the region of the lumbar vertebrae. The lumbar vertebrae are five in number (see chapter 4,

the section on the skeleton and the spinal column) and correspond to the Five Principles and to the five basic planes of the life of each person, namely: the couple, the family, the job, the home, and the country (or region).

When we are going through a period when we are having trouble accepting or integrating changes that are taking place, the lumbar vertebrae can express the unconscious fear of these changes. This is often because such changes upset our habits and our reference points, and that is often difficult for many people to accept without getting uptight, which is exactly what happens with lumbago. Lumbago can also speak about difficulties accepting things that have been brought into question, especially in the familial and professional arenas, or about difficulties changing our position or attitude in a relationship.

▸ SCIATICA

Sciatica is a pinching of the sciatic nerve where it leaves the spinal column in the lumbar area. It corresponds to lumbago in terms of its meaning; however, there is a supplementary precision to this condition. While lumbago is a locale-specific pain that speaks to us of an overall feeling, sciatica is a pain that travels and can even move around from the spinal column right down to the little toe. Sciatica is a more precise feeling that expresses difficulties clearing and letting go of old patterns. Sciatica follows the path of the Urinary Bladder meridian, which manages the clearing of old memories. Therefore, it's a question of tension linked to accepting change on one of the five life planes: the couple, the family, the job, the home, and the country (or region). The tension is caused by a difficulty in letting go of old beliefs or habits, old patterns or modes of thought, or places where we once found a certain balance and material or psychological support.

▸ VERTIGO

Vertigo is a sensation of loss of balance, of having the earth give way underfoot or of seeing orientation points we count on as being stable start to "dance." Vertigo expresses a need to be in control of the space surrounding us and a search for precise, defined, stable points of reference. This is why it mainly concerns anxious people or those who seem detached. One of the essential tools of balance in the body are the ears, particularly the inner ear, which is responsible for our sense of physical stability. So the ear, which belongs to the Water element, represents our fundamental orientation and reference points in life. With the fear of not being able to master what might happen, the space around us is dizzying. In some cases this directly involves a certain physical environment, such as vertigo in high places. In other cases it can be a situation that provokes vertigo. The classic case is vertigo felt on rides in amusement parks or during the practice of sports in which our spatial orientation points are disturbed, something I have found to be the case in the practice of aikido.

▶ WEIGHT ISSUES

Issues around body weight are signs of material or emotional insecurity in relation to the near or distant future. They also mean that we are having difficulty integrating those times in life when we encounter lack or shortages. With weight issues we are usually talking about an insecurity that is unconscious, a fear of lack that is not recognized; however, the person feels a need to stock up "just in case." Another type of insecurity manifesting as a weight issue is in relation to the external world. The fear of having to come to terms with the external world, risking not being able to do so, and of feeling destitute in the face of that can also lead a person to stock up, to "put some thickness between the world and me," to protect oneself with an eiderdown of flesh or fat. Overweight people are very often tender and fragile souls in great need of reassurance. A more insidious and serious form of weight gain represents an attempt to denigrate oneself or punish oneself. Doing so allows us to devalue our own self-image to conform to some deeply held belief that says "You see that you're no good—you're ugly and people can't love you." In this case the person seeks to make an image that is ugly to confirm the belief that he or she is unworthy of love.

Behind these three levels of meaning there is a common thread: the relationship with the mother (i.e., food) is out of balance and we are seeking to compensate. When this unbalanced relationship to food is particularly severe, bulimia or anorexia become supplementary ways of accentuating the message. **Bulimia** is the compulsive and sometimes uncontrollable need to eat food, immediately followed by regret to such an extent that the person might intentionally vomit in order to eat again or in order to not gain weight. This is a serious condition that is linked to depression and other serious side effects. Bulimia speaks about the need to fill an existential void, to control one's anxiety around food. Food represents the first connection to life and to the first being who loves us and gives us life and love—the mother. The relationship that we maintain with food is strongly impregnated with the memory of this relationship with the mother and the satisfying and compensatory role that she was able (or unable) to play. Every tension, frustration, lack, or need to compensate gets done with food. Fear, the uncertainty of not being able to begin again leads to a compulsive and repetitive attitude or to stocking up on food by eating to excess, and then purging.

Anorexia is the reverse phenomenon but essentially the same issue. Anorexia is characterized by a low weight, fear of gaining weight, a strong desire to be thin, and extreme food restriction. The emotional relationship with the mother and her representation as provider of sustenance was unsatisfactory. An absent mother (for one reason or another she was not available), one who didn't express love, someone who didn't want the child (or who wanted a girl instead of a boy or a boy instead of a girl) are the kind of deep-seated memories that sometimes devalue a person's relationship with food and lead to thinking that it is not attractive or worse, repulsive. Here too, anorexia can have serious consequences.

Infirmities and Handicaps

Infirmity is defined as "the quality or state of being; the condition of being feeble." The subject of infirmity is too complex to be resolved in a few lines, but it is, I believe, important to bring some understanding to the various conditions that fall under this heading. The suffering these issues entail are such that speaking about them a little can at least help us see them as not some form of misfortune or a fated injustice, but instead as a challenge, albeit one that is excessive, crazy, painful, or unfair.

Infirmity is written into the axis of choices at the time of incarnation. Among the structural constraints we choose for ourself in carrying out our Life Path, certain ones are sometimes hard or unpleasant. We can be born into a country, a family, a culture, or an era that might be easy or difficult based on our need for experimentation. Being born into a body with infirmities or acquiring an infirmity through an accident is part of the dynamic of choice. Yet life is not a punishment, and I reject the idea that we've come here to pay for our mistakes (refer to chapter 1 on the Earlier Heaven and the nonconscious, pages 11–15). Infirmities are not *punishments* but rather *handicaps,* and the meaning of these two words is fundamental to understanding because in the case of punishment it means we are not "good," and in the case of handicap it means that we are "strong." Because who is given a handicap in sports? Those who are clearly the strongest! Life is not vicious or perverse— it gives to each one according to the abilities of that person, and if it entrusts us with arduous tasks it is because it knows that we are capable of surmounting them (but also because we need them). Life knows how to offer us challenges that lead us into moving through them, always knowing how to tailor them to our abilities. And when I say "life" I am thinking "us," because it is we who have chosen the handicap in the Earlier Heaven, in our nonconscious.

Infirmities at birth are then karmic memories coming from the Earlier Heaven, whereas accidental infirmities are the choice of the nonconscious. These infirmities are always life challenges chosen by strong, powerful beings. This perhaps helps us better understand the discomfort that is often present in the way those in good health look at those who are infirm—especially those in good health who spend their days complaining about their own lives.

Among the lessons that life has sent my way there is one that will be engraved in me forever. One day I was walking down a street at a time when I was undergoing some mild difficulties that I had allowed to disturb me. As I walked along I was mulling over my black thoughts when my glance met that of a little girl coming my way who sent me a radiant smile as our eyes met. I was pierced through and through by a searing emotion because this little girl of eight or nine was black (like my thoughts) and handicapped in both legs (and my problems were relational). She was walking with crutches as she held herself up on two bent legs, and the picture she presented to me, when she had every reason to doubt the beauty of life, was radiant with the joy of life and light. What a slap in the face, what a lesson, as in a lightning flash I came to understand the language of life and its message! So who was I then to dare lament my own life? This is a lesson that those with infirmities provide for us constantly. I regularly receive a catalog of the work of a group of disabled people who paint with their mouths and feet because they don't have arms and sometimes no legs either. The paintings and objects they make are always filled with life, simplicity, love, and hope.

Infirmities are incarnational choices to be overcome by those who have made these choices, but they are also opportunities for growth for all of us who are in good health. They are there to teach us all love, tolerance, acceptance, and humility.

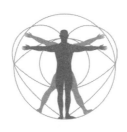

Conclusion

Until today becomes tomorrow, we will not know the benefits of the present.

CHINESE PROVERB

The conclusion that I want to give this book is really more like an introduction. My fondest desire is that this book will be for each reader an introduction to life and to having confidence in this life through the different way of looking at things that I am suggesting. Realizing that something is speaking to us through our body and that nothing happens by chance can frighten us or make us believe in fate. It is in fact just the opposite, and we must understand, as Paulo Coelho's alchemist said, "If Heaven gives us knowledge of the future, it is in order that it be changed." If life communicates intensely with us and expresses through our body what is wrong, this is so that we might change it.

All evolution in a human being begins with an awareness of what he or she is and what he or she does. This fundamental and necessary step is initiated by understanding the messages that come from the inner master or guide. However, this is not sufficient in itself. It would be simplistic to reduce someone's or one's own suffering to a statement such as "It's for such and such reason and it's because he chose to live this way." This would negatively reduce a particular health problem to a fatalistic attitude in the person's conscious plan, rendering the person unable to work at changing his deep, unconscious memories. The responsibility of each person in facing incarnation's choices and in facing life in general is not grounds for any kind of commentary. Conformity to the "law of life" is not to be judged by anyone, because no one knows its intimate details. May each one of us do the work set at our own doorstep, and the world will be in better shape.

Taoist monk Mencius said, "The great failing of men is in abandoning their own fields to go and remove the chaff from the neighbor's fields." This statement corresponds to seeing "the mote that is in thy brother's eye" but not "the beam that is in thine own" (Luke 6:41). In other words, it's a lot easier to see faults in others and give them unwanted advice than it is to acknowledge our own faults and do the hard work of changing ourselves. We make the error of focusing too much energy on others, trying to change them or taking it upon ourself to do something to "help" them when they haven't asked for help. Our priority should be to take charge of the life that has been entrusted to us. In managing it better, our presence increases on its own. In this way we can change the world.

Simply having awareness is not enough to miraculously have issues in the body disappear when we think we've understood what the soul is trying to say. This awareness must always be followed by the work of awakening and deep and sincere reflection on our behavior and our position in life. Then all we can do is bring about the changes that are necessary (and sometimes painful) to free up the energy that has densified in us, making us suffer. As well, we must accept the messages that come to us. We must accept their meaning, avoiding absolutely any possible confusion between being alert in listening to ourself and our body, and instead dwelling on listening—minus the follow-through.

Dwelling on listening means seeking out the body's cries for help and feeling sorry for ourself. It means taking the pain and suffering that accompanies the cries and making them a way of life, so that we identify with our pain. This perverse use of pain and suffering, a sign of a lack of affection and an infantile search for recognition, allows us to be pitied and looked after by others instead of taking the initiative to change.

Being alert in listening to ourself and to our body means being ready to receive messages from our inner master and changing or doing what's necessary to grow up and take responsibility for our state of health. The result of this is that pain and suffering will less and less be a part of our life. We will have less and less of a need to talk *about* ourself because we will be better able to communicate *with* ourself. Our exchanges with the outer world, less taken up by the clearing of tension, stress, or emotions, will then become more and more enriching and impregnated with truth.

The path is sometimes long and arduous before we are able to successfully engage the process of liberation that turns everything around and leads to healing. Quite often, others (friends, doctors, psychologists, therapists, spiritual guides) can help us and even sometimes treat us. However, we are the only one who can truly heal ourself. The healing can be simple and fast if the symptoms are benign, and more difficult if the illness is deep or considered incurable. It always depends on our deeply seated decision as to whether or not we want to heal. This decision, taken well beyond any conscious intention, belongs to each one of us. Our sincere belief in our ability to make it through can help us a great deal in the work of liberation. The final element, ultimately, is something indefinable, tucked away in the deepest part of ourself and whose fabulous power often shows up because it makes miracles every day: Life . . .

The following figure summarizes the mind/body interaction as delineated in the previous chapters. You will find in it all the major symbolic axes of the various parts of the human body, and you will then have a simple way of finding the meaning of the issues of the soul that impact the body.

To be pondered and kept safe inside of yourself like an opening, a

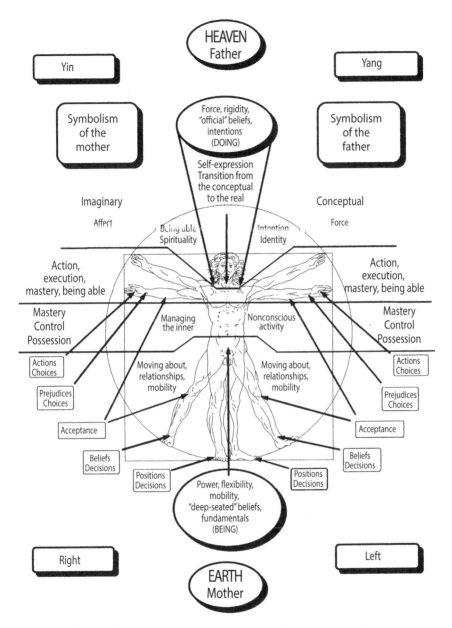

The body/mind strata: lateralization of the somatizations
in the human being

beacon, on the sometimes bumpy road of life. Bon voyage to each one
of you!

Index

Numbers in *italics* indicate illustrations.

Books of Related Interest

Overcoming Acute and Chronic Pain
Keys to Treatment Based on Your Emotional Type
by Marc S. Micozzi, M.D., Ph.D., and Sebhia Marie Dibra

Your Emotional Type
Key to the Therapies That Will Work for You
by Michael A. Jawer and Marc S. Micozzi, M.D., Ph.D.

The Science of Planetary Signatures in Medicine
Restoring the Cosmic Foundations of Healing
by Jennifer T. Gehl, MHS
With Marc S.Micozzi, M.D., Ph.D.

Emotion and Healing in the Energy Body
A Handbook of Subtle Energies in Massage and Yoga
by Robert Henderson

The Inner Cause
A Psychology of Symptoms from A to Z
by Martin Brofman
Foreword by Christian Tal Schaller, M.D.

The Miracle of Regenerative Medicine
How to Naturally Reverse the Aging Process
by Elisa Lottor, Ph.D., H.M.D.
Foreword by Judi Goldstone, M.D.

Natural Remedies for Inflammation
by Christopher Vasey, N.D.

You Are Your Own Best Medicine
A Doctor's Advice on the Body's Natural Healing Powers
by Frédéric Saldmann, M.D.

INNER TRADITIONS • BEAR & COMPANY
P.O. Box 388
Rochester, VT 05767
1-800-246-8648
www.InnerTraditions.com

Or contact your local bookseller